The No B.S. Alkaline Diet

By: Felicia Gordon

CONTENTS:

Introduction: --- 5

    The Basics -- 5

    What makes food alkaline or acidic? ----------------------------------- 7

    What are the Benefits of the Alkaline Diet? ------------------------- 8

    How to Get Started on the Alkaline Diet --------------------------- 13

    How to monitor the pH level of the body? ------------------------- 18

    The Best Alkaline Diet -- 21

The Best Alkaline Foods: -- 23

    Foods That Reduce Body Acid -------------------------------------- 23

The Acid Alkaline Balance Diet --- 37

    How Acids Affect the Glycemic Index ---------------------------- 37

Specifics of Alkaline Cooking -- 39

Alkaline Shopping --- 43

Alkaline Diet for Weight Loss --- 49

Alkaline Ash-Producing Foods -- 56

Alkaline Recipe Box: --- 62

    Breakfast Recipes -- 62

        Easy Pumpkin Patties --- 62

        Delicious Halloumi and Carrot Patties ---------------- 64

        Coconut Chia Strawberry Pudding --------------------- 66

        Simple Tofu Scramble ---------------------------------- 68

        Healthy Quinoa and Apple Breakfast ---------------- 70

        Healthy Avocado Breakfast Salad -------------------- 72

    Lunch Recipes --- 74

        Easy Chickpea and Kale Mash ---------------------------- 74

        Quinoa and Kale Salad ----------------------------------- 76

        Delicious Cauliflower Tabouli -------------------------- 78

        Spicy Honey Tofu -- 80

        Spicy and Tasty Tuna Salad ---------------------------- 82

        Sweet potato and Zucchini Fritters -------------------- 83

Quick and Simple Egg and Avocado Salad ------------------ 86

Dinner Recipes -- 88

Roasted Vegetable Pasta ------------------------------------ 88

Yummy Egg Stuffed Cucumber ----------------------------- 90

Delicious Marinated Eggplant --------------------------------- 92

Crispy Tofu Steaks -- 94

Healthy Sautéed Leeks and Cabbage ---------------------- 96

Salmon with Mushroom and Spinach ------------------------ 97

Tasty Veggie Quinoa Patties -------------------------------- 99

Simple Lemon Wild Salmon ------------------------------- 101

Crustless Cheese Spinach Quiche ------------------------- 103

Healthy Tomato and Spinach Frittata -------------------- 105

Quick Sautéed Shallots with Carrots --------------------- 107

Tasty Tomato and Carrot Soup ---------------------------- 108

Quinoa Stuffed Bell Peppers ------------------------------ 111

Yummy Sweet Potato Soup -------------------------------- 113

14 Day Alkaline Diet Meal Plan ----------------------------------- 115

Day 1 --- 117

Day 2 --- 118

Day 3 --- 118

Day 4 --- 118

Day 5 --- 119

Day 6 --- 119

Day 7 --- 120

Day 8 --- 120

Day 9 --- 120

Day 10 -- 121

Day 11 -- 121

Day 12 -- 121

Day 13 -- 122

Day 14 -- 122

Turmeric Ginger Lemon Detox Tea ------------------------------- 123

Wild Garlic Pesto --- 123

Raw Pad Thai --- 123

Gazpacho--- 124

Spinach Frittata: -- 124

Shopping Lists -- 125

Buy Organic When Possible -- 125

Knowing the Alkalinity of Soil --------------------------------------- 125

Drink Alkaline Water--- 125

Complete Alkaline Diet Grocery List --------------------------------- 126

Foods to Avoid on an Alkaline Diet --------------------------------- 127

Additional Habits that Cause Acidity in the Body----------------- 128

Conclusion --- 129

Introduction:

What is the Alkaline Diet All About:

The Alkaline diet is also called the alkaline ash diet, acid ash diet, alkaline acid diet, or acid alkaline diet. This is actually a group of diets loosely related to each other. The main idea is that there are certain foods that directly affect the pH and acidity of the body's fluids, such as the blood and urine. This effect is believed to be therapeutic for certain health issues.

The Basics

The body has its own regulatory mechanism for balancing pH or its acid-base condition. The alkaline diet claims to help or boost this function. The traditional concept of the alkaline diet is to avoid eating poultry, meats, grains and cheese. The goal is to make the urine less acidic and more alkaline. This means increasing the urine's pH level. This is believed to help prevent the recurrence of UTIs (urinary tract infections) and discourage the formation of kidney stones (nephrolithiasis).

When eating foods, the body burns them to extract calories or energy. The extracted energy will then be used by the cells. If not, then some of these will be stored. This burning process is a slow and well-controlled one. So, when something gets burned, a residue is produced. It's like burning wood and ash is left behind. This ash is classified as either alkaline or acidic.

The Alkaline Diet was developed with the help of the US National Institute of Health as a means to lower blood pressure without the need for medication. Aside from being able to lower blood pressure, the Alkaline Diet has also proven to lower the risk of other diseases such as stroke, heart failure, diabetes, cancer, osteoporosis, and kidney stones. Not only will it work for you today, it's designed in such a way that it will have long term effects—so you can be sure that you'll be able to live a long and healthy life.

The Alkaline Diet is comprised of low-fat or non-fat dairy, fruits, vegetables, lean meats, whole grains, poultry, fish, beans, and nuts that are filled with various vitamins and minerals such as potassium, magnesium and calcium that your body certainly needs to develop and function. It is a diet that is high in fiber and low in fat so it would be easy for you to lose weight and lower your cholesterol levels and it also aims to reduce the amount of sodium that you consume so the systems of the body can be stabilized. This way, you can live your life the best way possible. Aside from eating the right kinds of food, it is also recommended that you lessen or quit smoking and exercise regularly so you can be sure that you'll be able to maintain your ideal weight and that a lot of diseases can be prevented.

If you choose to follow the ALKALINE diet, your systolic blood pressure will be able to drop by at least 7 to 12 points, which is a big help for your cholesterol levels to go down and make sure that you would not be suffering from any heart ailments or strokes anytime soon.

According to the diet, the acidity or alkalinity of the ash will have an effect on the body. Acidic ash will cause the body's fluids to become more acidic. Alkaline ash will cause the body's fluid pH to become more alkaline. Eating foods that produce neutral ash will have no effect on the body.

Acid ash is believed to increase the body's vulnerability to certain diseases. Alkaline ash is considered to have protective effects on the body. By eating more alkaline ash-producing foods, the body becomes "alkalinized" and health improves.

What composes the alkaline diet?

Recognized as a diet that most Hollywood celebrities love, the Alkaline Diet is said to help a person lose weight and also avoid certain diseases such as cancer, heart ailments, arthritis and Alzheimer's Disease. The said diet also keeps muscles and bones strong, making you a more active and reliable individual. It is also very beneficial when it comes to losing weight the right way in a short amount of time.

This is because the diet gets rid of some kinds of meat, processed foods, refined sugar and wheat that let your body produce the bad kind of acid which is not healthy for you. Meanwhile, if you eat the right kinds of food, then you can be sure that you'll be on the path to good health—and the Alkaline Diet has basically everything you need to be on the said path.

It is said that if you lessen the intake of acidic foods, then your body will not easily be susceptible to diseases and you'll be more active and energetic. It's also a way of cleaning up both your mind and body. In summation, the Alkaline Diet makes use of more meat and protein, and less carbohydrates. This is mainly because meat and protein were the staple foods of hunter-gatherers. However, one has to make sure that he gets to avoid trans fats, and omega-6 fats, because these wouldn't work well with the diet.

According to the diet, different kinds of foods have different effects in the body. Meats, grains, poultry, eggs, fish and cheese produce acid ash in the body. Vegetables and fruits, with the exception of plums, prunes and cranberries, produce alkaline ash. The designation of alkaline or acid ash depends on the effect of the food residue after combustion happens and not on the actual acidity of the food.

For example, citrus foods are known as acidic but in the alkaline diet, these are considered alkaline-producing foods because the residue has an alkalizing effect in the body.

The components of food determine whether the residue becomes acidic or alkaline. Components such as sulfur, phosphate and protein will leave acidic ash residue. Food components like calcium, potassium and magnesium will leave alkaline ash residue.

Food groups considered as acidic, neutral or alkaline include:

Acidic food group: eggs, dairy, fish, poultry, meats, alcohol and grains

Neutral food group: natural fats, sugars and starches

Alkaline food groups: nuts, vegetables, legumes and fruits

What is the body's pH and how is it regulated?

The body's pH refers to how acidic or alkaline the body fluids are. The pH range is:

Acidic: pH 0 to 6.99

Neutral: pH 7

Alkaline: pH 7.11 to 14

In the body, different fluids have different pH levels. It isn't uniform. For instance, the stomach is naturally acidic, even if there is no food. It becomes more acidic around mealtimes, contributing to the feelings of hunger. The acidity comes from the stomach acids, particularly HCl (hydrochloric acid). The normal stomach pH is 2 to 3.5, a highly acidic condition. Acidity is not always a bad thing in the body. The highly acidic environment of the stomach is necessary for digestion because it aids in breaking down tough food components.

The blood, on the other hand, needs a more alkaline environment. It normally has a pH of 7.35 to 7.45, which is in a slightly alkaline range. The blood pH has to be within the normal range at all times. If not, the cells will cease to function properly and a whole lot of serious health problems will develop. If the pH range is not within these values, there could be serious problems. If left untreated, it can turn fatal. However, problems with blood pH only happen as part of disease conditions. The food does not directly affect blood pH.

Thankfully, the body has an effective pH balancing mechanism called the acid-base homeostatic process. This involves the respiratory system and the metabolic system (gut). If the blood pH is acidic, the respirations speed up and the gut slows down to retain more base or alkaline compounds. If the blood pH becomes too alkaline, the respirations slow down and gut movement speeds up to lose more base or alkaline compounds. The urine also plays a part in balancing the blood pH.

What the foods affect is the pH of the urine. This is what the alkaline diet targets.

What makes food alkaline or acidic?

The pH of food in the alkaline diet depends on the pH of the residue once all its components are burned by the body. The most vital rule is that high alkaline foods are those that contain large amounts of alkaline minerals such as potassium, magnesium, sodium and calcium. However, even if a food does contain large amounts of these alkaline minerals, it may still be considered acidic if it also has any of the following:

- Sugar, especially added sugars and refined white sugar

- Fungi, such as mushrooms

- Yeast

- Fermented, such as soy sauce

- Processed, refined or microwaved

These standards explain why it is surprising to see certain acidic foods classified as alkaline in this diet plan. For example, fruits are considered healthy but are classified as acidifying because most of them have high sugar content. The sugar has an acidifying effect in the body. Another example is banana. It is an excellent source of the alkaline mineral potassium. However, it is classified as acidic food because it has about 25% sugar. Other fruits like lemon, lime, avocados and tomatoes are generally thought of as acidic foods, but in the alkaline diet, these fruits are classified as alkaline because these have low sugar.

Sugar is an important determinant in the alkaline diet. The blood can deviate from its normal pH range in the presence of too much sugar. This is a recipe for a double disaster. Too much sugar is a major factor in the development of diabetic condition and all its complications. The excess sugar load in the blood will acidify it and cause even more problems. This is a potent combination that can cause serious chronic health problems such as diabetes and cancer.

The longer this process continues, the more problems arise. These health problems will also become more serious and harder to treat, and all it takes is to simply adjust intake and concentrate on eating more alkaline foods.

What are the Benefits of the Alkaline Diet?

The primary benefit of following the alkaline diet is that it restores or at least brings the body's pH from acidic to more alkaline. Too much acidity can produce lots of health problems and an alkaline diet can help prevent these.

Other benefits of following the alkaline diet go beyond the prevention of symptoms and problems related to too much acid. The alkaline environment helps tissues to function better.

Better energy

Cells must function well in order for the body to produce and use energy well. Acidity interferes with proper cellular processes and reduces energy levels. By going alkaline, the cells can function better. More energy will be produced and the other cells will have more to use for their own functions. This will result to higher energy levels.

Better gum and dental health

If the body is too acidic, the oral cavity is also acidic. Acidity will cause the dental enamel to erode, which will promote the formation of dental carries, plaques and cavities. This is also among the leading causes of bad breath. The acidic environment in the mouth promotes the overgrowth of bacteria. This will cause several oral health problems such as various gum diseases. This will also increase the risk for tooth decay. Most people notice improvement in their breath and overall dental health once they go on an alkaline diet.

Better immunity

When the various cells in the body are healthy, the immune system functions better. The integrity of the cells is great. Cellular integrity protects the cells from infections. The pathogens will find it difficult to enter and cause trouble. If the pH in the body is low (acidic), the cells will find it hard to keep their structures intact. This will allow toxins and pathogens to easily enter and cause more damage. These pathogens and toxins can easily get inside the cells and alter it. This will stimulate the development of health problems. Cancer, for instance, starts off this way. This is also a major reason why some people more frequently get colds and other infections compared to those who follow the alkaline diet.

Reduction in inflammation and pain

Magnesium is an important mineral in the body. It also has a vital role in maintaining the body's pH balance. If the body becomes acidic, the cells will release their magnesium stores to help in neutralizing the acidity. The more acidic the body, the more magnesium is required to counter its effects. This may be ideal but magnesium does not only function for acid neutralizing. The body has so many other uses for magnesium. Using a lot for acid neutralizing can seriously deplete the resources for the other tissues and cellular processes to use.

One of the major tissues affected is the joint. Low magnesium in the body is one of the factors that cause joint diseases and inflammatory conditions. Also, inflammation in the other tissues in the body is also attributed to low magnesium stores. Eating alkaline foods that are also rich in magnesium can replenish the resources and have more for the cells to use.

It strengthens the Neurons

When neurological processes are restored and protected, you get to protect yourself from Alzheimer's Disease and memory loss. Degenerative diseases could also be prevented.

This happens because alkaline foods also contain L-Theanine, an amino acid that promotes better neurological health—and not a lot of food products are able to do this.

Better Weight Control

This is a culmination of all the positive effects of alkalinity in the body. The cells function better, so that energy is better distributed. Fats are used properly and the body has enough energy. This will reduce cravings and hunger cues. That means reduction in the frequency of hunger cues and better appetite control. Fats and energy are also burned much more efficiently, reducing the risk of accumulating more fats that contribute to weight gain.

Preventing Stomach Upset

Thermogenesis, the term given to fat to energy conversion, is increased by at least 8 to 10 % when someone uses alkaline foods in his daily diet. This not only burns fat, but also regulates the digestive process.

Alkaline foods also reduce intestinal gas, and could also prevent certain diseases from happening, such as ulcers, ulcerative colitis, and Crohn's Disease.

Slower Aging Process

The aging process is driven by the damage to cells. When cells easily degrade and repair is slow, the aging process is accelerated. If the cells are able to repair damage efficiently and at a faster rate, the aging process slows down. In an acidic environment, the cells get easily damaged and at a much faster rate. Repair is slowed in acidic pH. In an alkaline environment, cells do not get as much damage and when any injury gets repaired sooner.

Also, the aging process is accelerated due to oxidative stress. This is caused by the accumulation of free radicals and toxins that eat away at the cells. Acidic pH in the body supports oxidative stress. Alkaline pH helps in reducing the toxin load and oxidative stress. These promote younger-looking, healthier cells that give a younger appearance.

Perfect for Athletes

This is mainly because they know that if they eat too much fat, their bodies would suffer, and their hearts would grow weaker—and that's never a good thing because they live such active lives.

More so, when you adhere to these diets, it would be easy for your body to turn nutrients into ketogenic energy. When you have ketones in your system, you get to perk yourself up, and you have enough energy to get through the day—and help you out with whatever it is that you have to do!

Avoiding Chronic Inflammation

Chronic inflammation is the reason why so many diseases are contracted. These diseases include Type 2 Diabetes, Various Heart Diseases, and Cancer. Many believe this happens because grains are—you guessed it—inflammatory.

Staying away from Auto-Immune Diseases

Take a look at it this way: Gliadin, also known as the worst kind of gluten, is actually responsible for affecting the pancreas, thyroids, and the entire immune system by means of releasing antibodies that aren't meant to get out yet. When these antibodies go out, auto-immune diseases can be a risk and one may be afflicted with diseases such as Hashimoto's Disease, type 1 diabetes, and hypothyroidism, among others.

Incidentally, research has shown that Alzheimer's Disease is often triggered by high-grain diets. It releasers blockers in the brain that could break mental processes down, and therefore lead to the deterioration of the brain.

Develop a Healthy Gut

Doctors believe that the state of your gut could affect the state of your brain. After all, when you're hungry, you tend to make decisions that are not well thought out.

As you can see, your gut is in charge of a lot of things in your body—which we often fail to see in our daily life. These things include the way you utilize fat and carbohydrates, nutrient absorption, feeling satiated, and vitamin/neurotransmitter production. It can also affect your levels of inflammation, detoxification, and immunity against diseases. (This is not an exhaustive list, these are just some of the factors that stand out).

This is also because of the vagus nerve, found in the gut, which is the longest of the 12 cranial nerves. This is the main channel between your digestive system, and your nerve cells that send signals to the brain.

In short, it's absolutely vital to take gut health seriously since it impacts almost every other facet of our physical health (and one could even argue that it impacts our mental health as well.) Why? Well, because if the given processes above do not work right, you might be afflicted with certain medical conditions, such as dementia, diabetes, allergies, cancer, ADHD, asthma, and other chronic health problems.

Also, when your gut is healthy, your brain gets to make more serotonin—the hormone that keeps you happy and keeps your sanity in check. It's a much better regulator than most anti-depressants.

Avoid Vitamin-D Deficiency

Even if you consume Vitamin D in supplement form, it actually depletes inside the body pretty fast, and acid makes that depletion even faster. Moreover, WGA, or Wheat Germ Agglutinin also causes bacterial growth that kills Vitamin D and damages the gut—and could do much worse to your body in the future.

Dehydration Will Be Prevented

Unlike coffee and soda, alkaline beverages make amazing drinks because they keep the body hydrated. Alkaline food has moisture, as mentioned in an earlier chapter, which means that it actually has water, unlike other flavored or carbonated drinks.

You're on the Road to Feeling So Much Better

It sounds cheesy, sure, but the thing is when you adhere to these diet combination, it's like you're giving yourself the chance to feel good again.

These days, people go through a lot of things. Their lives—possibly yours, too—could turn nasty in just a second, and it would be even harder if they don't take care of their health. So, as early as now, you should consider this book a chance for you to reverse your health—for the better, of course!

Top Health Benefits from a well-balanced pH in the body

- Skin has better elasticity and looks more radiant and youthful

- Sleep is deeper and more restful

- Abundant physical energy

- Reduced frequency of suffering from colds, flu viruses and headaches

- Improved digestion

- Reduced symptoms of arthritis

- Reduction of overgrowth of yeast (*Candida* infection)

- Reduced risk for osteoporosis

- Improvement of mental acuity and better mental alertness

Safe, healthy, legal natural high from better hormonal and neurotransmitter levels

How to Get Started on the Alkaline Diet

To start the alkaline diet, prepare yourself for a lifetime of dietary changes. It is not a short-term, one-time only diet, even though this is how most people view the term "diet". It is a long-term decision. Knowing the right foods that produce the desired healthy benefits will greatly help you succeed in making your body more alkaline.

Change how you view food

The very first step is to change the way you look at and treat food itself. Take this time to evaluate yourself. Is food merely for sustenance? Is it merely a source of calories? Or is it a source of energy and materials that the body can use to be healthy?

Food should not just be a source of energy. If this is your view, you are likely to be not too concerned on quality. Rather, it's more on quantity. The right thinking should be on the quality of food. The alkaline diet teaches you to be more aware of the things you eat and how they ultimately affect the balance in your body. What are the ingredients in food? Do they supply the body's nutritional requirements? Do they contain potentially harmful components? What is the body's reaction to the various components of food?

Also, never think that diets are just about counting calories. It's important is that you supplement your diet with exercise.

Get a list of the different types of alkaline foods and how they affect the body. A comprehensive list is available at the end of this book. Use this list as a guide on what to include in meals, what to limit and what to avoid.

Drink lots of pure, clean water

Water is vital for normal functioning of the various tissues. In fact, about 70% of the body is composed of water. It is used as a medium for various cellular processes. It is also used to dilute salts, toxins and other substances to keep them under control. Water is used as a medium for excreting wastes and toxins. It is crucial to replenish water stores in the body because it can be easily depleted through sweat, tears, urine, feces, etc.

As the human body is made up of 75% water, it comes as no surprise that a person needs to be able to sustain that amount. If a person loses water in his system, he will be dehydrated and this is dangerous for your physical health. Because of this, it's important to understand how vital water is for you and how much of it you need per day. Water also aids in weight loss. Because it has no preservatives and is not carbonated, it doesn't add any calories or carbohydrates to your body, which is essential for people who want to lose weight.

Surprisingly, water nowadays is acidic. Try to test various commercial bottled water brands and you'll see they are acidic. The usual pH range would be as acidic as pH 4 to 6. Drinking lots of water is good, but not if it's acidic. It will only add more acidity inside the body. Choose clean, pure water. If possible, get spring water, with all the natural dissolved minerals in it. Distilled water in bottles is already stripped off of all the dissolved substances that are beneficial to the body.

Sometimes, the weather gets too hot that a person may feel dehydrated. To prevent being sick or experiencing heat stroke because of extremely hot weather, it's important that a person drinks 13 to 15 cups of water per day or that he eats fruits that are loaded with fluids, too. Aside from water, a person with fever or diarrhea may also have to take oral supplements or sports drinks to replenish the loss of water in his system. You can also try fruits such as watermelons or pears—they're pretty much filled with water and that's why they are good for you.

Also, if you are fond of working out or of any activity that makes you sweat then you certainly need to drink a lot of water to make up for what you have lost. You need to add 1 to 3 more cups to your usual intake.

Aside from water, you could also drink the following:

- **Coconut Water.** Coconut Water is dubbed as nature's own sports drink that has a thermogenic effect and helps make sure that the gut is strong and safe.
- **Juice.** Not the processed kind, though. Try to make your own green juices (with vegetables as base) and mix and match ingredients. It's actually fun, and you'd also help yourself gain a lot of nutrients by doing so, too. Try using the following: *cucumber, celery, beet, carrot, ginger, parsley, spinach, and cabbage.* Then add either of the following: *berries, watermelon, aloe vera, goji berry, acai berry, etc.*
- **Shakes and Smoothies.** Shakes and smoothies are fine, as long as you made them yourself, and they do not contain additives.
- **Tea.** Herbal teas, as you may know by now, are important parts of your diet. Make sure you do not add sugar or milk, though. 3 to 5 cups per day is already good.

The lack of dissolved substances makes distilled water more acidic than regular, clean water. Instead of getting distilled water, choose filtered water. It still retains some of the valuable dissolved materials and is less acidic.

Make various meals out of cruciferous vegetables

Here's the thing: the more alkaline foods you eat, the more weight you'll lose. When you chew alkaline foods, it automatically means that you are already burning and digesting your food—and of course, it's only natural that you get to chew these vegetables, especially if you eat them instead of your usual snacks or fatty foods, in general. If you want to eat your snacks, you need to have the mindset of eating a whole bunch of cruciferous vegetables first—so later, you'd only eat a small amount of the snacks.

Cruciferous vegetables come from the Cruciferae Family. These are vegetables that are generally cultivated for food production. Interestingly, the name also originated from "Cruciferae", which in early Latin literally means "cross-bearing", an allusion to the shape of the flowers that seem to resemble crosses. Prime examples of cruciferous vegetables include: *Brussels sprouts, bok choy, garden cress, broccoli, cabbage,* and *cauliflower.*

These vegetables are known to be essential parts of the Negative Calorie Diet because they are high in cellulose, water, and Vitamin C, together with essential phytochemicals and nutrients that the body needs.

Most cruciferous vegetables also contain glycosylates that are said to prevent cancer, drive toxins away from the body, and could suit the taste of many—and that's why they are used in most plant-based recipes!

You see, your overall calorie intake will ultimately be reduced when you eat alkaline foods instead of high-calorie ones—and if you exercise as you do so, you'd really see substantial amount of weight loss.

Once you start the diet, you'd really notice that you are losing weight. Over time, though, you might feel a lack of energy—but then you'd also realize that as your metabolism slows down, it would then work to provide you with more energy—which will then be used by your body as fuel to live!

What you should keep in mind, though, is that you have to eat at least every 2 to 3 hours—so you can sustain the energy that your body needs, and you also have to take note that you cannot eat sugar or honey—and other sugar replacements, with the exception of Stevia. It's also important not to use any artificial dressings because more often than not, they contain sugar. For dressings, you could use garlic or Dijon mustard mixed with yogurt and your choice of herbs.

Evaluate food on hand

Most of the time, there isn't any real need to throw everything that's already in the fridge or pantry and buy new kinds of food. There are no specialized food requirements for the alkaline diet. It's actually a simple type of diet, utilizing the common everyday food items. Check whatever is on hand and compare them to the list. If there are acidic foods, which is highly probable there will be, there's no need to throw them out. A great thing about the alkaline diet is that foods can be mixed to make a healthier dish.

Mix acidic foods with alkaline foods to balance out the acidity. For instance, herbs are a great way of balancing the pH of meals. Mix ginger with beef to even out the pH. Add curry spices to chicken to reduce its acid-forming effect. Not only do herbs balance the pH, these are also excellent at adding more flavor to meals. Another example of mixing foods to balance the pH is by wrapping bacon around asparagus sticks and then grilling or steaming them. Drizzle healthy alkalizing oils over acidic foods to improve the pH. The omega-3 fats from these oils will help create a more alkaline environment in the body. Be creative. There is no need for specialized food items.

It would also help you to be on the lookout for macronutrients, also known as macros. These measure your daily intake of carbohydrates, protein, and fats. The amount that you should take might be different from everybody else's, so you do have to know exactly where you stand. For this, you have to understand that it would be important to know your measurements, starting with the size of your waist. To know the accurate size of your waist, go get a tape measure. Then, find the widest point around your belly button, and measure from there—and not from where you have placed your belt at. Then, go ahead and learn what your real weight is by weighing yourself first thing in the morning—without any clothes on.

Once you know that, you have to enter your body weight in lbs and in kilograms, and you also have to know what your body fat percentage is. If you have no idea what your body fat percentage is, you could keep the following in mind:

- **10-14%.** This is usually called the beach body look. Muscles and fat may be separated, but you may not see it in every muscle group. There might also be veins on the arms and legs.

- **5-9%.** This means that there's a lot of vascularity in the muscles—think body builders, or athletes, especially those who wrestle or play football, boxing even. The abs would also be well-defined—which means body fat is pretty low.

- **15-19%.** With these percentages, you could expect that there is less vascularity and that muscles are also not that defined anymore. You could see a great separation between them—except for the arms.

- **20-24%.** This is another common type of body fat percentage. The muscle and fat separation is almost non-existent, and the muscle groups are also not strained or vascular.

- **25-29%.** This is already considered obese, at least, for men. This is because it's obvious how the stomach is already round, and that the waist has also increased or has widened. Neck fat may also be there, but veins and muscles may not be visible.

- **30-34%.** This means that the hips are smaller than the body and waist—too much fat is visible.

This way, you would know the right portions that can help you—which you'll learn more about in Chapter 6.

Learn to listen to "hunger cues"

Pay attention to how you feel and if you know you're already hungry, go ahead and eat something, but try to scale it out. For example, ask yourself if you really are hungry in a span of 1 to 10, 10 being the highest. By questioning yourself, you'd know if you actually should eat already, but again, do not starve yourself. This helps you separate actual physical hunger from emotional hunger. Often we think we're hungry, but we're just bored or want to be comforted and so we turn to food.

Start slowly

To avoid getting overwhelmed with all the changes in following the alkaline diet, start slowly. Incorporate 2 to 3 alkaline meals per week. There is no need to totally change your entire week's menu just to follow this diet plan. You can start slowly as you gradually replace whatever acidic foods you have at present with more alkaline ones. Slowly add more alkaline recipes until you have at least 10 to 20 different alkaline meals per week. These meals should be tasty, so you can still enjoy the foods you want. Again, the key is to balance acidic with alkaline foods. This way, you can also curb any cravings that will come as you make the transition to a full alkaline diet.

How can you make better food choices to improve pH?

Food choices are the cornerstone to improving and balancing pH levels of the body. Everything ultimately depends on what foods were chosen to become part of each and every meal, including snacks. Making the right choice every time is not always easy. To get through the tougher times, live by these guidelines:

- Choose white meat over red meats. Healthier meat alternatives also include meat substitutes and seafood.

- Choose wild rice or yeast-free bread instead of fries or rolls.

- Choose almond milk instead of cow's milk.

- Choose sparkling water instead of alcoholic beverages.

- Choose vegetables as main dishes instead of starches or meats.

- Choose to fill the plate first with plant foods like vegetables, grains and fruits so that there is little space left for acid-forming food items.

- Choose vegetables with dips or fresh grilled fruit instead of prepackaged or processed snacks.

- Choose to use cold-pressed olive oil for cooking instead of butter or saturated fats.

- Choose to have dressings, sauces and condiments on the side instead of having them already mixed into the food when eating out or ordering take-out.

- Choose to exercise every day, like walking for at least 30 minutes instead of watching a 30-minute TV show.

- Choose to reduce the stress levels by performing yoga, meditation and other similar relaxation techniques.

How to monitor the pH level of the body?

The simplest and easiest method of monitoring acidity in the body is by checking the urine pH. This is not a requirement to be successful but it helps immensely in checking how well the body responds to the diet. Urine pH monitoring can help in tailoring the diet according to your body's needs. Some people can restore alkalinity by just adding more alkalizing vegetables. Some may need to make huge cut-backs in their meat consumption. Responses are different among individuals and the change is a personal thing. To make the alkaline diet more suitable for your needs, monitor urine pH levels to evaluate your body's responses.

Testing is done every day. Early morning urine is the best sample that can give more reliable results compared to random urine sampling throughout the day. There are ready to use test strips available in pharmacies that you can use to test urine pH levels from the comfort of your home. These test strips can give reliable pH readings without having to take the urine sample to laboratories or medical clinics.

To use the urine pH test strip:

- Remove the test strip from the package. If the test kit comes in a roll, carefully tear off a 3-inch piece.

- Sit down on the toilet bowl and start to urinate. Catch the midstream urine for the test sample. The first few ml of urine (the first 2 seconds worth of urine) is more acidic than the rest and is not the most reliable sample. Readings will give a false positive result. This means getting a very acidic urine pH that's not an actual representation of the entire urine pH. The higher acidity readings is a result of sitting and getting more concentrated in the urinary bladder compared to the rest of the urine.

- Once in midstream, take the urine test strip and place it directly under the stream of urine. Hold it there until the strip is thoroughly moistened.

- Take the test strip then compare it immediately to the chart that comes with the test kit. Match the color of the moistened test strip with the keyed color chart printed on the side of test bottle or of the packaging.

- The number that best matches the color of the test strip will be the urine sample's pH level.

- Record the result. Use this for future reference.

- Discard used test strip properly. These strips are not reusable.

- Testing the urine pH can be done as often as desired. However, once per day is enough to gauge the body's pH level for that day.

Be Consistent

Don't try to lose weight today and then go ahead with your bad eating habits again next week. What's important here, as well as in any kind of diet, is consistency. You have to make sure that you are committed to it and that you don't give in to temptation. For this, it would be nice to keep a food journal and make sure to fill it up with information regarding what you just ate and add some healthy recipes—like those you'll find in this book!

How to make correct substitutions from common acidic foods to more alkaline choices?

To make meal more alkaline, reduce the amount and frequency of acidic foods. There are alkaline substitutes available for common food items that you can use to enjoy tasty meals, beverages and snacks while balancing the body's pH.

Acidic Food	Substitute with
Butter	Clarified butter; cold-pressed olive oil
Flour	Almond flour or skinless almonds finely crushed
White rice	Basmati or wild rice
White potatoes	Sweet potatoes
Yeast breads	Sprouted grains
Yeast	Lemon juice and baking soda
Soda	Sparkling water
Coffee	Herbal tea
Creamer	Almond milk
Canned fruits	Frozen fruits, no additives
Gelatin (made from meat or animal parts like knuckles)	Agar-agar (made from seaweeds)
Condiments	Fresh spices and herbs
Sugar	Clover honey, Stevia
Peanuts	Chestnuts, almonds
Navy beans	Lentils

Whole eggs	Egg whites
Red meats	Firm tofu, poultry

The Best Alkaline Diet

You can reduce the body acid. If you have cancer, arthritis, heart disease, stroke and other health conditions your body is acidic. The sign of acidity in the body and whether it is in the blood or body tissue is the acidosis. The pH level is the determining factor between your health and development of diseases.

When cancer patients are tested, they are found to have extreme pH acidity and depletion of oxygen in the cells which encourages development of the cancerous cells. This can form stomach cancer, colon cancer, liver cancer esophagus cancer, pancreatic cancer and other types of cancers and diseases.

Which are the alkalizing foods?

An alkaline diet is mainly composed of fresh fruits and vegetables, certain low calorific whole grains, nuts, seeds, oils and many other foods which we have listed to make it easy for you to consume them regularly.

The ideal alkaline diet involves balancing of acidifying foods and alkalizing foods to a ratio of 20:80. The body through its organs like the liver and kidneys neutralizes and eliminates any excess acids from the body. However, even a healthy body has a limit as to how much acid it can neutralize and eliminate through the body systems effectively.

Excessive acidity strains the body systems as they try to detoxify these acids. Naturally, the body is created in a way that it makes it able to maintain the acid-alkaline balance on its own provided that:

- you consume a well-balanced alkaline diet

- the organs function properly

- *excess acidity in the body is avoided*

This is one of the ways to remain healthy and energetic naturally. Unfortunately, the main diet in many homes is comprised of foods that cause acidity in the body. These acid-forming foods strain the detoxifying system so they accumulate in the body.

The body mechanisms become overwhelmed with the work of removing excess acids from the body. You need to eat an alkalizing diet that will reverse the acidity and reduce the strain on the organs like the kidneys and the liver.

The following are the high alkaline foods. Raisins and spinach are among the most alkaline foods.

Alkalizing Vegetables

Beets

Broccoli

Carrots

Cabbage

Cauliflower

Celery

Collard greens

Cucumber

Kale

Lettuce

Onion

Peas

Pepper

Spinach

Zucchini

Alkalizing Fruits

Apples

Bananas

Grapes

Lemon

Lime

Melon

Peach

Pear

Orange

Watermelon

Alkalizing Carbohydrates

Stevia

Maple syrup

Rice syrup

Fresh corn

Amaranth

Wild rice

Potato skins

Alkalizing Proteins

Almonds

Chestnuts

Goat's milk

Hazelnuts

Soybeans

Tofu

Tempeh

Alkalizing Herbs and Spices

Basil

Cinnamon

Garlic

Ginger

Mustard

Thyme

Fats

Olive oil

Flaxseed oil

Canola oil

Avocado

The Best Alkaline Foods:

Foods That Reduce Body Acid

Different parts of the body have different pH levels. The stomach is very acidic. The acid in the stomach is there to help it to digest different types of foods. The effect your food has on your body whether acid-forming or alkaline-forming, does not depend on the pH of the food. That is why fruits like lemons and limes which are expected to promote acidity within the body are alkalizing because of the citric acid in them.

The best alkaline meal plan to reduce body acids should include the following alkaline foods.

Almonds

Almond nuts and almond milk are alkaline foods which are among the world's healthiest foods. They are alkalizing foods which you can eat to reduce body acids and maintain a natural pH balance. Almonds lower cholesterol, increase muscle gain and are rich in protein, calcium, dietary fiber and iron. They can be eaten between meals as a snack or used as an ingredient in alkaline meal plan diets. A few almonds are enough to give you these benefits and neutralize the body acids.

For each 100g:

- Protein – 44%

- Calcium – 27%

- *Iron – 25%*

Asparagus

Asparagus is a top food in the alkaline list that helps to neutralize the acidity on the body. This is grouped among the strongest alkaline foods. It is also packed with vitamins, antioxidants, detoxifying and anti-aging properties.

That is why you should start adding it to your meal plan to gain these benefits and reduce body fluids.

For each 100g:

- Vitamin A - 15%

- Iron – 12%

- *Vitamin C – 9%*

Avocado

Both avocado and avocado oils are packed with nutritional benefits putting them at the top of the list of super-foods as well as one of the best alkaline foods. Avocados are rich in healthy fats, fiber, Vitamin C, Vitamin A and potassium.

You can substitute avocado oil for acid-forming oils. Avocado supplies the good fats in the diet that fight the bad fats in the body. Make dips or slice the avocado and eat it raw.

For each 100g:

- Fiber - 27%

- Vitamin C - 17%

- *Vitamin A - 3%*

Basil

Herbs and spices play an important role in making us alkaline by cancelling the effects of acid-promoting foods. Basil is a great alkaline addition to most menus although you may not have known. It is also rich in flavonoids and is a good source of Vitamin K and Vitamin A. Add basil to your list of alkalizing foods. Vitamin K helps in the clotting of blood.

For each 100g:

- Vitamin K – 345%

- Vitamin A – 175%

- *Calcium – 18%*

Beetroot

Not only is beetroot alkaline, it has anti-cancerous properties and is a rich source of iron, folate and carotenoids. Many people eat beetroots as a side dish but you can make a healthy juice or smoothie with them. It is an important antioxidant and that is why it fights cancer in the body.

For each 100g:

- Folate - 75%

- Vitamin K - 11%

- *Vitamin C - 8%*

Broccoli

This is one of the alkaline foods that you should take often because of its nutritional value and its ability to fight and prevent some types of cancers. Broccoli boosts your pH level which in turn reduces acidity in the body.

Many people eat broccoli almost daily but 3-4 times a week is good enough. Steam the broccoli to get the most benefits from it. You can also bake it or use it in the broccoli recipes as a healthy addition to your alkaline meal diet. The high Vitamin C content helps to fight infections and diseases including cancer.

For each 100g:

- Vitamin C - 135%

- Vitamin A - 11%

- *Calcium – 4%*

Brussels sprouts

Brussels sprouts are healthy vegetables belonging to the same family as broccoli and cauliflower which break down body acids in the body leaving you more alkaline.

For each 100g:

- Vitamin C - 142%

- *Vitamin A - 15%*

Cabbage

Cabbage is known to fight and prevent cancer and that is why it should be eaten often. In fact, some studies show that it can aid in reversing some types of cancer especially if it is organically grown. It is low in calories and makes you feel full. It helps in digestion and boosts your pH levels.

You should steam this alkaline vegetable lightly on low heat, so that it retains the nutrients which would otherwise be destroyed by too much cooking, but still tastes great! Look for a good recipe for cabbage and you will enjoy it.

For each 100g:

- Vitamin A – 54%

- Calcium – 5%

- *Vitamin C – 3%*

Carrot

Carrots are rich in Vitamin A, Vitamin C, antioxidants, fiber and potassium. Carrots are good for the eyes whether you consume them as a juice, smoothie, steamed or when used in salads or chewed raw.

They are alkaline and tasty and add color to the food. Many people have a good habit of including carrots as part of their diet but what they don't know is that it is one of the best foods to eat because of their vitamin, carotenoid and flavonoid content. Start chewing a raw carrot now and then or include them in your alkaline diet.

For each 100g:

- Vitamin A - 336%

- Vitamin C – 10%

- *Calcium – 3%*

Cauliflower

Cauliflower is rich in Vitamin C and a non-fruit source of this essential vitamin. It can be steamed or eaten raw in salads or smoothies. You can also mix it with other ingredients to make an alkaline diet that fights cancerous diseases and other illnesses and diseases.

For each 100g:

- Vitamin C – 77%

- Calcium – 2%

- *Iron – 2%*

Celery

This is one of the alkaline foods that you can use to make salads, smoothies or soup whether you like the taste or not. Celery is one of the world's healthiest foods so you get used to eating it often. It is a low-calorie vegetable which is packed with nutrients.

You can use it to make a green smoothie or add it to a fruit smoothie. It is recommended to people with osteoarthritis, rheumatoid arthritis and cancer.

Collard Greens

These strong alkaline vegetables are among the most effective cancer-fighting foods you can find. They are so rich in Vitamin A and other nutrients that you cannot afford to leave the out of your alkaline meal plan.

For each 100g:

- Vitamin A – 230%

- Vitamin C- 20%

- *Calcium – 20%*

Eggplant

Eggplant is a popular veggie you should always add when you go food shopping. This is one of those foods you are sure to find in many diets. You can eat as many times as you like without worrying about calories. You can eat it several times a day either as a side dish, roasted or cooked with your food to balance the acidity in other foods consumed each day.

Flaxseed and Flax Oil

Consuming freshly ground flaxseed or whole seeds as well as cooking with flax oil will help your body to stay alkaline. You can add whole flaxseeds in your meal plan or sprinkle them on food. Try to add them to your smoothies or ingredients when preparing your meals.

For each 100g:

- Calcium – 37%

- *Iron – 46%*

Garlic

Garlic is a powerhouse of so many nutrients and also a body cleanser used in detoxifying diets. Garlic lowers blood pressure, aids in fighting and preventing cancers. Adding some cloves of garlic to your green cleansing smoothie or adding minced garlic while cooking is a good habit. Adding garlic to onions while stir-frying your favorite alkaline vegetable adds a great taste to them. Each clove consists of about 2% of Vitamin C. Garlic has anti-bacterial properties so it is used to fight infections.

Ginger

The health benefits of ginger are numerous and people have realized this so they are using it more and more. Ginger is one of the superfoods that you don't want to miss in your alkaline diet. It is alkaline and it has anti-inflammatory and detoxifying properties.

You can mince or grind the fresh garlic when cooking it or make ginger tea.

For each 100g:

- Protein – 44%

- Calcium – 27%

- Iron – 25%

Goat's Milk

Goat's milk is alkaline and it is better than cow's milk by far. Cow's milk is acidic on the body while goat's milk is alkalizing on the body. There are many people who are lactose intolerant but they have goat milk tolerance.

For each 100g:

- Calcium – 33%

- Vitamin A - 10%

- *Vitamin C - 5%*

Grapefruit

This is another superfood which you can enjoy. It is one of the most alkaline foods that you should include in your alkaline meal plan. Although it may have an acidic taste, when you consume it, the effect is alkalizing on the body. Grapefruit boosts your body's metabolism.

For each 100g:

- *Vitamin C – 73%*

Green beans

You will find green beans in many grocery stores since they are one of the most popular vegetables used in many household. Green beans are alkaline and low in calories. Preparing and cooking them is quite easy and you can find them in many recipes.

You can enjoy green beans as a side dish, stir-fried or mixed with other ingredients to make stew. They are a good source of Vitamin C, fiber and potassium. You can also get some amount of calcium and iron from them.

For each 100g:

- *Vitamin C – 30%*

Herbal Teas

The black tea most people are used to drinking is acidic on the body. To have an alkalizing effect, you need to start drinking herbal teas.

Herbal teas such as ginger, ginseng, artichoke, hibiscus, chamomile and cinnamon teas among many others do not contain caffeine. They have medicinal benefits which make them popular among users. They are therapeutic and they contain antioxidants and have a pleasant fragrance.

Kale

The health benefits of kale are numerous. Kale is an alkaline food which is a rich source of Vitamin K, Vitamin C, Vitamin A, fiber and a bit of calcium. You should consume kale regularly to boost your immune system because of the high Vitamin C content. The Vitamin A they provide is also high for your eyes and other nutritional benefits while Vitamin K helps in the clotting of the blood.

Adding kale leaves (without the hard stem) to your green juices or smoothies, salads or steaming and eating them as a side dish adds value to your meals. You can add the kale to green leafy vegetables like baby spinach and puree them in a blender until smooth.

For each 100g:

- Vitamin A - 206%

- Vitamin C– 134 %

- *Calcium – 9%*

Kiwi

Kiwi is an alkaline fruit which you can enjoy.

Leeks

Leeks come from the onion family and they are an alkaline food. They rate highly as a pH booster just like onions while they are rich in Vitamin A and Vitamin C. Leeks are popularly used in soups but you can also steam them and add them to other vegetables to take as part of your alkaline diet.

Lemon

Many people believe that lemon is acid-forming because of its acidic taste but this is not so. When lemon is consumed it becomes alkalizing and it boosts your pH scale. Lemon is a good source of Vitamin C which neutralizes free radicals.

You should consume lemon for protective benefits against infections and some types of cancer like colon cancer. It also helps to detoxify the body of toxins. You should consume it regularly by squeezing it in your drinking water, adding a slice to your detoxifying water or using it as an ingredient in your recipes or take it as a lemonade beverage or cocktail, marmalade, jelly or as pickles.

Lemon helps in throat infections, indigestion and constipation, skin care, toothaches, weight-loss, relieves respiratory problems, controls high blood pressure, removes wrinkles, dandruff, corns, old scars and blackheads, sooths toothaches and heals fever and colds.

For each 100g:

- *Vitamin C – 51%*

Lentils

There are many varieties of lentils which you can add to the table. Lentils are alkaline when you consume them. They are rich in iron, fiber, vitamins, minerals and other nutrients.

Lettuce

Although some people believe lettuce has no nutritional value, it does. By eating it you get an alkaline response in the body. Even if you do not eat it for real sustenance, you should eat it for the alkalizing effect it has on the body.

Lima Beans

Lima beans are a good source of iron, calcium and Vitamin C. they are popular among vegetarians and vegans, they are rich in Vitamin C so you can take them even when you are not consuming citrus fruits.

Lime

As much as lime is acidic, it has an alkaline response to the body and it is good to add it to water for detoxification or add it to your green juice or smoothies. Lime raises your pH level when consumed so you should add it to your alkaline meals. Lime has many benefits like assisting digestion, detoxification, weight loss, respiratory problems, skin care, constipation, fever and other conditions. Lime is consumed as a beverage, pickles, jam, jelly and cocktail or in other forms.

Mango

Mangoes are a top food in the alkaline list. They are grouped among the strongest alkaline foods and are also packed with vitamins, antioxidants, detoxifying and anti-aging properties. That is why you should start adding them to your meal plan to gain these benefits.

Melon

Melons are alkaline but you should eat them alone without mixing them with other foods since they pass through the stomach fast. You will see why in later chapters.

Mint

Adding mint to your recipes gives you and you alkaline advantages. It is good to flavor your food or smoothie with this alkaline-forming food—indeed better than many other acid-forming spices and artificial flavorers.

Olive Oil

Olive oils have gained popularity for those who care about their health. There is virgin oil and extra virgin oil among other varieties. One Tablespoon of olive oil consists of 9.8g polyunsaturated fat and 1.4g monounsaturated fat.

Onion

Onion is an alkaline food that helps to neutralize the acidity on the body whether it is eaten raw or fried to make food dishes. This is grouped among the strongest alkaline foods and is also packed with vitamins, antioxidants, antibacterial and anti-aging properties. You should eat fresh onions more often because of their alkaline effect.

For each 100g:

- *Vitamin C – 17%*

Oranges

Oranges are popular fruits and they are among the world healthiest foods. They are packed with healing phytonutrient compounds which are mainly in the peel and white pulp. They are excellent sources of carotenoids and flavonoids. Oranges fight cancer, cardiovascular diseases and can help in preventing kidney stones as well as lowering blood pressure and cholesterol.

The antioxidants in oranges and other foods help to fight free radicals that cause cancer and other diseases. Eating oranges boosts your alkaline level since they are one of the most alkaline foods. They are packed with nature's antioxidants like Vitamin C which fight free radicals in and around cells so they do not destroy DNA and cause diseases like cancer.

They have a high Vitamin C content and you should consume them to boost your immune system as long as you don't mix them or other acidic foods like lemon, lime, pineapple, cucumber or grapefruits with your carbohydrates.

The digestion of acidic fruits is different from the digestion of carbohydrates. Oranges are also a good source of fiber, Vitamin A, Vitamin B1, folate, potassium and calcium.

Papaya

Papaya is packed with nature's carotenoids which helps the body fight diseases. This is a top food in the alkaline list that helps your body neutralize the acidity caused by consumption of acid-forming foods. Papaya is packed with vitamins, antioxidants and other health benefits. There are different types of papayas which you can enjoy throughout the year.

Parsley

Parsley is used to garnish chicken, steak and other foods. It is an alkaline spice which you should add to your vegetables when you go shopping. You can add it to your blender or juicer when you are preparing juice or smoothie to give it that refreshing taste.

You can grow parsley easily in your garden, pots or containers so you can have it ready and fresh when you need it. Use parsley to garnish your food.

Peas

Peas are a good alkaline food addition to your recipes. You can use them to make stew and other dishes or eat them as a side dish. You don't need to add butter to them because they have their own natural taste and the butter makes them acidic.

There are many dishes that you can make using peas. There are also so many stew recipes that you can get. Peas add color to your food.

For each 100g:

- Vitamin C - 97%

- *Vitamin A - 22%*

Pepper

Pepper whether green, red or yellow are alkaline when eaten and they boost the pH level. You can take eat them raw or you can stir fry them with olive oil, onions and garlic, add them to your recipes or make a vegetable salad. Peppers are a rich source of Vitamin C and other antioxidants and eating them regularly boosts the immune system. To stay alkaline, add peppers to your alkaline diet and you will reap multiple health benefits.

For each 100g:

- Vitamin C - 200%

- *Vitamin A - 11 %*

Pumpkin

There are many pumpkin recipes which you can use to make colorful alkaline dishes. It is packed with antioxidants that fight diseases like cancer.

For each 100g:
- Vitamin A - 171%

- *Vitamin A - 17%*

Raisins

Raisins are rich in Vitamin C. These are one of the foods with the highest alkaline content and you should eat them to boost your pH level.

Soybeans

Many people know the health benefits associated with soybeans and soybean products such as tempeh, tofu, and soy milk. You can substitute meat with tempeh and soy milk with cow's milk if your aim is reducing body acids from your systems. Of course Tofu makes a great meat substitute also.

For each 100g:

- Iron – 162%

- Vitamin C – 19%

- *Calcium – 52%*

Spinach

If you think of the best sources of alkaline-promoting foods, spinach is one of them. Spinach is among the strongest alkalizing foods that should be added to your diet, especially raw spinach. If you don't like it raw then steam it lightly or stir fry it with onions. Raw spinach can be consumed as a salad, a smoothie or juice. Buy baby spinach and put in the blender and add other vegetables like cucumbers, kale, lettuce and celery to make green juice.

For each 100g:

- Vitamin A – 56%

- Vitamin C – 14%

- *Iron – 4%*

Squash
Just like its counterpart the pumpkin, squash is an important alkaline food packed with vitamins, minerals and antioxidants. The carotenoids in squash and pumpkin give them their color.

Sweet potato
Sweet potatoes which are alkaline in nature are rich in antioxidants which fight diseases like cancer. You can roast, bake, stew or boil sweet potato or use it as an ingredient in many tasty diets.

Instead of cooking potatoes which are acid-forming unless they are cooked with their skin on, incorporate sweet potatoes in your alkaline meal plan. Consume them for breakfast instead of acid-forming foods like bread and oats.

They are tasty and even kids like them. Sweet potatoes are available in orange, white, purple and other varieties. You can buy them fresh in many grocery stores and farmers' markets.

For each 100g:

- *Vitamin A – 369%*

Tomato
Tomatoes are rich in lycopene, Vitamin A, Vitamin C and other carotenoids. You can use tomatoes to make sauce, dips, salads, burgers, sandwiches, smoothies, juices and as an ingredient in many recipes.

Many dishes prepared in many homes use tomatoes as one of the ingredients. There are many varieties of tomatoes which include plum tomatoes, pear tomatoes, cherry tomatoes and grape tomatoes among others.

Watermelon
Watermelon is one of the most alkaline fruits you can enjoy. It is a top food in the alkaline list which helps to neutralize the acidity in your body. This is grouped among the strongest alkaline foods and is also packed with vitamins, antioxidants, detoxifying and anti-aging properties.

If you take them with other foods in one meal they cause fermentation to the other foods that are digested slowly. To gain maximum health benefits eat watermelon and other types of melons alone.

A watermelon juice is colorful and tasty. Cut it into big chunks and puree in a blender or juice extractor, pour into a glass and enjoy. You can take the juice cool or chilled by adding crushed ice cubes when making the juice.

Zucchini
This is an alkaline vegetable that is easy to grow and is also readily available in most grocery stores and farmers' markets. You can steam or bake zucchini or use it in the many recipes. You can grow zucchini in your garden since they are easy to grow and they take a short time to mature. This way, you can have them fresh when you need them.

The Acid Alkaline Balance Diet

What is the proper pH balance?

Enzymes or biological molecules within the body are usually proteins, although they may be in other forms. What we eat is broken down by enzymes which act as catalysts in the metabolic processes that sustain our lives. Enzymes cause and speed up chemical reactions in the body which include digestion among other functions.

Enzymes are very selective about which chemical reactions they will speed up. In the body, the way the enzymes behave is affected by the pH level in the body tissues and in the blood. That is why it is essential to maintain the right pH levels for a healthier you. If this is not done, the blood or body tissues may cause diseases which could have otherwise been prevented.

The acid alkaline balance diet is therefore crucial to our health and well-being. You need this diet so that the enzymes can digest the foods properly and promote the absorption of nutrients into the blood to be transported from one part of the body to another.

The acid alkaline balance diet helps the body's metabolism to carry out different functions effectively so that the body eliminates the waste products from the digestive system as it should instead of depositing them in different parts of the body.

The alkaline diet also preserves the sodium, calcium, magnesium and iron in the muscles and bones to prevent them from being offloaded by an alkaline-deficient diet.

This prevents diseases such as arthritis, osteoporosis, multiple sclerosis and lupus. The best alkaline diet promotes health and that is why you should adopt it.

How Acids Affect the Glycemic Index

The Glycemic Index or GI, is basically a guide that tells you how fast carbohydrates get into your bloodstream and turn into sugar, or glucose, which could affect the acidity in your body. There are free online calculators that would help you determine the said amounts but what this chapter will tell you about is how you can manage your GI to make sure that it won't be so high. If you take in a lot of calories, as in more than 1,600, your GI might go higher than usual—so it's best that you take control of that. Basically, what's important is that your body takes a long time to break down carbohydrates into sugar so your body won't be full of sugar and you won't suffer from various ailments. Here are some tips that will help you put your Glycemic Index under control:

1. Know that you can eat as many fruits and vegetables as you like. This is because fruits and vegetables are considered as "Water Foods", which means that they can do no harm to your blood sugar and won't contribute to worsening your situation. However, you have to avoid canned or preserved fruits or vegetables because there are preservatives used in them already and they'll only make your blood sugar levels higher.

2. Eat less-processed or unprocessed grains. No one's asking you to say goodbye to carbohydrates, but you do have to make sure that you eat only the right kinds. This means that you should concentrate on wheat berries, brown rise, millet, and kernel dough instead of rice. Muesli or Granola Breakfast cereals are also fine as long as they are using whole grains and don't contain added sugars and preservatives.

3. Coal foods. Coal foods in particular won't contribute much to your GI because they are high in protein and fiber. Some of the best examples include beans, whole grains, seafood, lean meats, seeds, and nuts, as well as whole-wheat pasta.

4. Avoid fire foods. While coal foods are low in GI, fire foods are very high and that's exactly why you have to avoid them. Some examples include sweet chips, white pasta, white rice, white bread and most heavily processed foods.

5. Stay away from starch. Starchy foods are not good for you because they contribute to your daily GI levels. This means that instead of eating those processed foods or chips for snacks, you should just eat fruits such as pears, papaya, berries, peaches, and apples because they're good for you and they'd add more water to your system.

6. Make sure that you chew your food well and that you eat slowly. When you're eating, you can take as much time as you want because if you chew your food well and if you're not eating in haste, it means that you will be able to avoid having a high Glycemic Index and at the same time, you'd be able to make your metabolic rate go faster, too. When this happens, you get to burn fat quickly and so you also make sure that your health is in tip-top shape.

7. And, find alternatives to the usual foods that you eat. There are days when you seem to crave for foods that aren't really good for you and would just spike up your blood sugar levels. What you can do is find an alternative and eat foods that are in the same category but would still keep your health in check. Check out the list below so you'll have a better idea of what this is about:

- Wild or brown rice instead of white rice.

- Whole wheat instead of regular pasta.

- Rolled or steel-cut oats instead of oatmeal.

- Raisin, oat, muesli, or granola instead of processed corn flakes or breakfast cereals.

- Mashed cauliflower, winter squash, yams, and sweet potatoes instead of mashed or fried white potatoes.

- Leafy greens or peas instead of corn.

- Bran flakes instead of cornflakes.

By following these tips, you can make sure that your Glycemic Index will be in check. In the next chapter, find out how you can still eat fats—even on an alkaline diet.

Specifics of Alkaline Cooking

Starting a new diet really isn't just about knowing the right kinds of food to eat, but also knowing the right ways to cook or prepare them, or to make substitutes when the situation calls for it.

Simple Cooking Tips

- You can't have Pasta, but you can always make your own pasta by using spaghetti squash, instead.

- You can make use of your leftover dinner as lunch for the following day.

- You can make one huge salad at the start of the week, and then make use of some of the ingredients for the rest of the week. Basically, you can mix and match ingredients—as long as you keep them fresh in the fridge! Of course you'll want to avoid putting any dressing on the salad until right before eating to keep the leaves and vegetables crisp.

- You can also cook meat in bulk and freeze it, or store it for the week.

- The adjustment period may take time. That's a given. But that doesn't mean that you have to give up if you don't change everything right away. Remember that every good thing actually takes time, so just hang in there.

- Omelets always work for breakfast.

- Never use same sifters from various flours. Again, doing so would prevent cross-contamination from happening.

- Never prepare gluten and Alkaline foods on the same surface.

- Never ever forget to read labels. These will help you understand whether what you're having—or adding to your meals—is Alkaline, or not.

- Make homemade broth to consume and use in cooking. It makes your immune system stronger, and you can always use the broth as base for your soups and stews, too.

- It would be best to have separate utensils for cooking Alkaline dishes only, and another set of utensils only for your Non-Gluten Free and non-alkaline meals. This way, cross contamination could be avoided.

- Don't use the same toasters for various kinds of breads.

- Don't cook and eat without moving. You have to aid the Alkaline Diet with some movement AKA exercise. Even simple brisk walking would do.

- Alkaline foods should never be deep-fried. If you're eating out, make sure to ask the restaurant staff about whether breaded and unbreaded products have been cooked in the same surface or not.

- Stick with it for at least 30 days. It's said that the Alkaline Diet works best if you learn how to stick with it for at least a month. At this rate, your body learns how to adjust to it, and would consider it a regular part of your life!

Use alkaline-friendly flours

These are:

- **Arrowroot Flour**. This is one of the best thickeners you can get out there and is actually tasteless when cooked.

- **Buckwheat Flour**. While it has wheat in its name, you can relax because it's not actually wheat. It's from the rhubarb family and would give your dishes a nutty flavor.

- **Brown Rice Flour**. This is bran-milled flour that has an earthy flavor and is best for making gnocchi.

- **White Rice Flour.** This may be a bit bland but gives your recipes a light and easy to eat texture.

- **Rice Flour.** This one has delicate texture when cooked and is great for making sponge cakes and noodles.

- **Tapioca Flour.** This is pretty chewy and is perfect for patties and casseroles.

- **Soya Flour.** Made from soybeans, this one has quite a nutty taste and is said to be one of the best alternatives to flour.

- **Quinoa Flour.** Quinoa is related to spinach and has been around for over 5,000 years. It works best for desserts, such as pastries and cakes.

Use alkaline substitutes

Make sure that the way you cook won't be detrimental to your health by learning how to make use of Alkaline Substitutes. For these, you can try the following:

Trail Mix. Trail Mixes could be fun with the help of alkaline chips, candies, dried fruits, raisins, and peanuts. Don't buy date trail mixes as they're usually rolled in non-gluten free oat flours.

Thickeners. For thickeners, you can use tapioca starch or arrowroot flour. Dry pudding could work, too.

Soy and Teriyaki Sauce. You can mostly use Liquid Aminos, which you can usually find at health stores. You could also make use of most Asian Sauces or choose to make your own teriyaki sauce by mixing soy sauce substitute with equal parts of wine and sugar, too.

Pie Crust. Basically, you could just turn crusted recipes into non-crusted ones. Say, quiche without the crust or something. However, if you're trying to make pastry, it would be best to just crush alkaline cereals or cookies and press them onto a greased pie pan. Bake the way you would a regular pie and you're all set!

Hot Breakfast/Oatmeal. You can mostly use corn grits. Fry them, and add sugar, cinnamon, or butter. Quinoa and Amaranth cereals could work, too.

Granola. You can make your own Alkaline Granola by tossing spices, seasoning, some oil, vanilla, honey, alkaline cereal, seeds, and nuts altogether. Bake at 300 degrees for around an hour and add dried fruits shortly before serving.

Flour. Alkaline flours, and Cornstarch could work. Amaranth is often the number 1 choice, but feel free to choose whatever you want.

Flour and Bun Tortillas. You should make use of rice wraps, available in most Thai/Asian stores. You can also use corn tortillas, alkaline bread, and lettuce. You can also use *Nori* for stuffing—just like you would with sushi.

Croutons. For croutons, you can make use of Alkaline bread mixed with Parmesan cheese.

Breading and Coatings. Make use of alkaline breadcrumbs, crushed potato chips, corn flour, or corn meal for your coating needs.

Binders. Make use of guar gum, xanthan gum, or gelatin.

Alkaline Shopping

Another thing that you have to understand about the Alkaline Diet is that it is essential for you to choose proper portions. When you portion your food, it becomes easier for you to make sense of what you're eating—and because of that, you can get more of the nutrients that you need, too.

Start with meat…and all kinds of protein

So, what should make up your portions, then? First, you can start with Protein, which definitely includes turkey or chicken breasts, salmon, tuna, halibut, pork loin or pork chops, non-fat mozzarella cheese, tofu, beans, lean beef, veal, soy milk, yogurt, nuts and seeds, eggs, and egg whites. Protein is one of the body's essential nutrients because it is very beneficial. It can repair and replace tissues, hair, blood, nails and even muscles and a person need to sustain the amount of protein in his system so that he would not easily be susceptible to diseases. For athletes, protein is important because it builds muscles instead of fat and keeps them sturdy and on their feet. Body-builders rely on Protein a lot, too. Protein is also considered as the building blocks of tissue, which means that it can also be considered as one of life's building blocks. Without it, a person will feel unhealthy and would not be able to function well.

The recommended amount of Protein always depends on your age, sex, weight and level of activity. Around 50 to 175 grams per day is generally good. This also means that you can eat at least 5 to 6 ounces of protein-rich food each day. Men also need more Protein than women. If a woman eats 6 ounces of Protein each day, a man has to eat 7 to 8. Adults also need more Protein than children and so do bodybuilders. A bodybuilder has to eat 6 to 9 grams of protein per every pound of his weight. Other active adults have to eat 4 to 5 grams of protein each day, too.

Lots of vegetables

Veggies should make up at least ¾ of your plate. Most vegetables have low acid content. Males need around 2 to 3 cups of vegetables daily while women need 2 to 2 ½ cups. The same level goes for fruits. However, the amount may change depending on the kind of activity you do, your gender and also your age. Take note that again, men need more vegetables than women and that if they are extremely active or if they do 60 or more minutes of physical activity daily, they would need 4 to 5 cups of vegetables and around 3 to 4 cups of fruits. Kids need around 1 to 3 cups of vegetables and 2 to 3 cups of fruits daily.

Vegetables help reduce the risk of heart diseases such as heart attacks and stroke and can also protect the body against certain types of cancer. Vitamin C aids against inflammation and helps wounds heal fast. Plus, it also protects the body against several types of infections. Vegetables are also great sources of essential nutrients such as Vitamin C, Vitamin A, Folate and Dietary Fiber. Fiber not only aids in weight loss but also cleans the systems of the body and rids it of toxins. Aside from that, it's also important in regulating bowel movement. When this happens, it will be easy for you to digest food and be able to get the nutrients you need from the foods you eat. Fiber heightens the body's metabolic levels, too.

As some vegetables are high in potassium, it means that they can lower your blood pressure, decrease the level of bone loss and can also help in lowering blood pressure, as well. Some vegetables that are rich in potassium include potatoes, sweet potatoes, lima beans, beet greens, lentils, soy beans, tomatoes, tomato products and kidney beans, as well. Vegetables are rich in fiber so they can prevent obesity and Type II Diabetes and can definitely aid in making you lose weight fast.

Vegetables also keep the skin healthy and radiant, and vegetables that are rich in folate are great for pregnant and lactating women. These vegetables give them a chance to produce healthier kinds of milk. Aside from this, Folate also provides the body with healthy red blood cells which means that you will not be easily susceptible to diseases and that you can absorb other nutrients easily. Folate also protects the body against certain diseases such as spina bifida, tube defects and acephaly that are easily gotten when the baby is still inside the mother's womb. As you can see, eating vegetables can help protect the baby and make sure that he gets out well and healthy.

To make portion control easier, you can make use of the following vegetables:

- **Lettuce.** Aside from extremely low amount of acid, what you can expect about lettuce is that no matter how much you eat of it, it still won't make you gain a lot of weight. Lettuce that contain the most nutrients are red leaf, purple, or dark green.

- **Brussels Sprouts.** What's great about Brussels sprouts is that they're loaded with fiber and phytonutrients that make you lose weight and that prevent cancer. Sure, you may not like them at first, but when cooked right, they actually taste amazing.

- **Beets.** What's amazing about beets is that although they are sweet, they actually do not contain sugar and they are also filled with fiber, antioxidants, potassium, folate, and iron!

- **Mushrooms.** Mushrooms are not just the favorite pizza toppings of some, they're also quite amazing because they could boost and protect the immune system as they contain fiber, B Vitamins, potassium, and loads of antioxidants! The best variants include Portobello, Shitake, and White, amongst others.

- **Turnips.** Turnips promise low glycemic index, which means you'll also be protected from diabetes, and is also one of the best sources of Vitamin C.

- **Spinach.** Another miraculous vegetable, spinach is quite flavorful. It contains Vitamin K, Folic Acid, iron, beta-carotene, and phytonutrients that help you lose weight and protect you against loads of diseases. It also prevents macular degeneration.

- **Zucchini.** Another favorite, zucchini is sometimes known as the "miracle squash" because it allows you to feel satiated—without filling you up with calories. It's also filled with Vitamin A!

- **Garlic.** Garlic is amazing because it strengthens the immune system and helps fight colds, together with most urinary infections. It has lots of antimicrobial and antiviral properties!

- **Kale.** One of those vegetables that are part of many diet regimens these days, Kale is a great superfood that prevents breast cancer and is also filled with lots of phytonutrients. Aside from that, it's also one of the best sources of manganese, folic acid, and most vitamins, as well.

- **Carrots.** They are so low in cholesterol and fat, which makes them a perfect part of this diet. They're also rich in beta-carotene and Vitamin A—essential nutrients that the body needs.

- **Celery.** What's great about celery is that it's filled with cellulose and it's considered a high-volume food—which means that even if you eat a lot, you won't get fat. It's perfect for those who are trying to have healthy pregnancies, and is also filled with folate, vitamin C, and vitamin A, among others.

- **Fennel.** This prevents winter coughs, boosts your immune system, and is filled with lots of vitamins and minerals, as well.

- **Radishes.** They aid in digestion because they contain lots of sulfur compounds, antioxidants, and folic acid, and has twice the amount of calcium that leafy vegetables have.

- **Pumpkins.** Pumpkins have many antioxidants, beta-carotene, and essential vitamins. It's also so easy to add to a lot of dishes, so it's a great part of any diet! It lowers blood pressure, as well.

Add some carbohydrates

Next, you also have to realize that carbohydrates are not actually *that* bad. In fact, you need a good amount of them in any healthy, balanced diet. Carbohydrates are important to your body when taken in the right amount. Carbohydrates are essential because they boost your mood and increase the amounts of "happy hormones" in your body; they keep the memory sharp; they are good for your heart and have the right amount of soluble fiber that you need. Eating 5 to 10 grams of carbohydrates daily can lessen the amount of cholesterol in your system by at least 5 percent, and; they help control the amount of fat in your body, making sure that fat gets turned into glucose—which your body could then use as "energy" or fuel to live.

For this, you can try quinoa, whole wheat pizza, barley, bulgur, or popcorn. Basically, the mount of carbohydrates that you need depends on your lifestyle. For example, people who are lean and who regularly work out need just 100 to 150 grams of carbohydrates per day. This means that they can eat all the vegetables they want together with some fruits and healthy starches such as sweet potatoes, oats and rice.

If someone wants to lose weight but still cannot give up carbohydrates, he is allowed to eat 50 to 100 grams of carbohydrates per day. This means that he has to eat plenty of vegetables, around 2 to 3 pieces of fruits and a minimal amount of starchy carbohydrates each day.

And, try some good fats

Unlike what you're usually told, fats aren't all that bad. The right kinds of fats are very good for you and necessary for a healthy diet. Good fats provide you with energy and also help your body absorb nutrients easily plus they can also control or stabilize the body's cholesterol levels so you can live a healthy and well-balanced life. You can always start with mono-unsaturated fats, or those that are found mostly in oils and certain types of food. They decrease the risk of heart diseases and also control an insulin and blood sugar level which protects you from diabetes. They also help you feel full and satiated, so small amounts of monounsaturated fats, when added to your food, can help you feel full longer.

Then, you also can eat some poly-unsaturated fats, or fats found in oils and plant-based foods that can control cholesterol levels and protect you against heart diseases and certain types of cancer.

And of course, you shouldn't forget about Omega-3 Fatty Acids, which are found in tuna and most seafoods and are good because they keep the heart healthy and can reduce the risk of coronary heart disease, artery problems and irregular heartbeats. These fats also aid in weight loss.

Fat intake depends on your age, gender and lifestyle. Generally, adults and less active women should take 1,600-2,000 calories each day while teenagers and very active women and active men should take 2,500 calories or less each day. Doctors also recommend a 2,000 to 2,500 calorie diet or 44 to 78 grams of fat per day for everyone as a total of all kinds of healthy fats.

If you're wondering where you could get healthy fats, here is a list of foods that are rich in healthy fats:

- **Seeds.** Seeds lower the amount of cholesterol in your body. Sunflower and Pumpkin Seeds are the best that you could try.

- **Peanut Butter.** This beloved sandwich spread is actually healthy for you because it is made up of mono-unsaturated fats. Choose finely ground ones instead of chunky/crispy ones with parts of nuts still in them. Choose natural peanut butter that hasn't been loaded with extra sugars. Now, you know that the classic Peanut Butter Sandwich can actually be good for you!

- **Omega 3 Fortified Foods.** Check labels of different food products and if you see that they are loaded with Omega 3, go for them. Oatmeal is one good example of this.

- **Olive Oil.** Use olive oil for cooking and you will be able to serve something healthy and good for the heart.

- **Nuts.** Nuts are also healthy sources of fats and what's great is that fats from nuts are good for the heart. Walnuts, Pecans and Hazelnuts provide you with ample amounts of nutrients. Make sure though that you don't eat them during every meal because it would be bad for your cholesterol levels. 1 ounce per meal per day would already be good. An ounce means around 35 peanuts, 24 almonds and 15 pecan halves. 18 cashews would also be good.

- **Kale, Spinach and Brussels sprouts.** These vegetables are good sources of omega 3 fatty acids that keep the heart healthy and can protect you against various diseases, as mentioned in an earlier chapter. 2 to 3 cups of these greens each day would be beneficial for you so don't forget to add them to your shopping list.

- **Ground Flaxseed.** This contains enough soluble fiber that can rid your body of toxins and that will certainly protect you against various diseases. It's also the reason why flaxseed is all the rage these days when it comes to diet regimens. Use flaxseed for cereals or salads and you'll be alright.

- **Fish.** As mentioned earlier, omega 3 fatty acids are examples of healthy fats and you can get those from fish such as sardines, trout, tuna, herring, mackerel and salmon. Aside from being full of healthy fats, they also aid in keeping your brain sharp and smart. 2 servings of fatty fish each week is essential.

- **Eggs.** Eggs are not only a good source of fat, it's a good source of protein, too. An egg per day would definitely keep the doctor away.

- **Beans.** Kidney Beans, Navy Beans, Soybeans and Lentils boost your mood and strengthen the body, too.

- **Avocado.** What's good about avocado is that you can make different dishes and dips out of it. Make a guacamole, salsa or add it in your omelets or sandwiches and you'll certainly enjoy it. It prevents osteoarthritis and is definitely good for the heart, too. A medium avocado per serving can be good for you.

Compute carb and protein intake

You also should compute your carbohydrate and protein intake, and make sure that it falls under 1.2 grams per meal or around 30 grams each day. For this, compute the following:

1. Daily Carb Intake (grams)

2. Daily Protein Ratio (grams/lb.)

When you make use of proper portions, it'll be easier for you to follow the alkaline diet.

Alkaline Diet for Weight Loss

When our bodies are too acidic, they adapt by creating more body fat in order to store the excess acid. Acidity deprives our bodies of vital nutrients and minerals. These are essential not only for healthy weight loss, but also for maintaining our energy levels. Without energy, there is nothing. Here are some really basic tips on how you can get started on the alkaline diet right away:

Drink more water

One of the reasons people have an unbalanced pH level is that they are poorly hydrated. In order to correct this, you should drink at least 2-3 liters of good-quality filtered water per day. This will also help your body flush out toxins in order to ensure better overall health. However, your fluid consumption should emphasize water, not other beverages such as caffeinated soft drinks, coffee, or tea, since these can increase your acidity. I am a really active person and I do lots of fitness. So, very often, I drink about 3 liters of water a day. In the summer, it's probably more than that. This is what works great for me, but everyone is different. I encourage you to experiment and figure out what works for you and for your lifestyle. People always tell me that I drink so much water that I am going to float away at some point!

I am sure you have already heard that drinking clean water is good for you, but are you actually in the habit of hydrating your body with good-quality water? Don't drink tap water. Use quality, filtered water. This is a very basic concept of Alkalinity, but it is very often overlooked.

Bottled water is not that beneficial because it contains many chemical ingredients that come off of the plastic bottle. I suggest you invest in quality alkaline filters and filter your water. I personally use an alkaline water pitcher with filters. These are great because you can always take them with you when you travel. They're a great investment, and I actually spend much less than what I used to spend on bottled water and energy drinks. Plus, I don't have to worry about toxins in tap water or bottled water. Besides, if you stick to buying bottled water, it can get really expensive in the long-term.

Water is also great for concentration. Yes! Many experts dedicated to memory improvement or rapid reading strategies recommend regularly sipping on water. If you feel thirsty, see it as a sign your body is sending you to tell you it is getting dehydrated. You should aim for prevention. Don't wait until you get thirsty. Make regular hydration one of your top priorities. You will feel so much better.

I like to throw in some fresh lemon juice or infuse my water with herbs and fruits. I also juice ginger (*really* alkaline) and make ginger ice cubes (I juice the ginger and freeze it into cubes). They are in the freezer, ready to grab and spice up my water and make it more alkaline.

I occasionally use green powders, especially alfalfa powder, and mineral salts. However, you must remember that your diet and lifestyle come first. Supplements can only enhance your healthy lifestyle, they will not create it for you.

Reduce your consumption of processed foods, which contain ingredients such as white flour and sugar

These foods may also contain preservatives, food colorants, and other unhealthy chemicals. Eating these foods can make your body more acidic, which in turn forces it to try to cope by pulling more alkaline buffers from different parts of your system. This can result in various health problems because important nutrients such as potassium, calcium, and zinc are lost. These foods are not natural; they are not what we were biologically designed to eat. Yet, people get addicted to processed foods. Do you know why? Many chemical ingredients are added into those foods in order to get the consumer hooked on them.

One of the biggest challenges I faced when switching to an alkaline diet was the fact that I had to reorganize my way of shopping. My old way was to go to my local supermarket once a week, pick all the sales and foods I liked, pack, and go back home. I was happy that I was saving time. Unfortunately, I was doing mindless shopping. After all, at the local supermarket I could buy everything in one go, but I would not focus on quality, which in the long run, results in more health, energy and even more time.

Now I no longer do it the 'quick supermarket' way. I know that in order to keep my alkaline lifestyle, I need to make sure my kitchen is always prepared and full of alkaline-friendly fresh foods. That is why I have a shopping schedule and I plan my shopping on a weekly basis. Grocery shopping plays a crucial part in my planning. Here's how I do it:

- Once or twice a week, I contact my local organic food store, which also gives me the option to shop online (a time-saver!). I order fresh fruits and veggies. They usually have discounts for regular clients, and I was surprised to see that their products were almost the same price as fruit and vegetables I would get from the local supermarket. Of course, it may depend on your country, state, and city. So, I encourage you to do some research so that you can support your local markets, save time, and choose the healthiest foods for yourself and your family. Real foods, yes! I am also a big fan of local organic markets.

- Once a month, I go to my local organic store and make sure to get stuff like: quality oils (olive, coconut, or avocado oil), raw almond milk (super alkaline!), coconut milk, healthy grains like quinoa or millet, herbs, spices, teas, legumes like chickpeas, lentils, and adzuki, and healthy nuts and seeds. I am also interested in trying some 'new stuff.' I am always willing to grab something I have never even heard of, then get back home, Google it, and find ways to cook it. This is how I learn all the time.

- Occasionally, I get seaweed like wakame or kombu. They can be easily stored in your fridge and are a great way to alkalinize your salads and soups. I occasionally buy natural food supplements, for example alfalfa powder or other powdered greens. I want to make sure my body gets enough minerals in a natural way.

I am a big fan of wellness on a budget, which is why I always try to pick up the best offers and discounts. Shopping in bulk is a great option, and so is proper planning. This is how you avoid temptations since there are only healthy foods in your kitchen. As they say, "Out of sight, out of mind." We definitely want to use this rule to make sure that the only foods on your mind are healthy, unprocessed, and alkaline foods.

Like I mentioned, in order to go alkaline, you don't have to go 100% vegan. Still, I encourage you to experiment and learn more about vegan alkaline cooking. Since the alkaline diet encourages reducing meat consumption, you should learn more about natural sources of proteins for vegans and vegetarians:

- Hemp (You can use hemp powder in your smoothies, it's really miraculous)
- Veggies (One cup of cooked spinach has about 7 grams of protein. Kale is pretty much the same.)
- Quinoa (It has about 9 grams of protein per cup.)
- Almond Butter (It is great with gluten-free breads and wraps. Two tablespoons of almond butter are about 8 grams of protein.)
- Other choices include: lentils (great in salads), and some occasional tofu or tempeh. I am not a big fan of tofu or tempeh, but I do use them in my recipes sometimes.

Many people are not successful with the alkaline diet and eventually quit because they try to do it against their nature. <u>They eliminate too many foods and try to survive on only green vegetables, giving up after a few days.</u>

I want to show you that the Alkaline Diet is not as restrictive as some say. It's all about finding balance and a nutritional lifestyle that works well for you. This is what this book encourages.

So, if you know that a 100% vegan lifestyle is not for you, don't worry. You can still do the alkaline diet by only reducing animal products as much as you can and adding more alkalizing foods. You can still live an alkaline life. So, let's move on to the next step!

Snack on fresh vegetables and nuts

In order to satisfy your hunger pangs, you can take fresh veggies such as carrots and celery and cut them into snack-size strips that you can dip in a healthy dip, like hummus. Extremely nutritious! You can supplement these with healthy alkaline seeds and nuts such as:

- Almonds
- Sunflower seeds
- Coconut
- Flax Seeds
- Pumpkin Seeds
- Sesame Seeds

Preparation is the key to success! I am almost sure that if you are reading this book, you have tried some kind of dieting before. Have you noticed that the worst part about dieting is what they tell you must be eliminated from your diet? How does that make you feel? Personally, I prefer a different approach.

Firstly, focus on <u>adding</u> some new, fresh, alkaline foods into your diet. Don't think about eliminating for now, but make sure that **you add new** delicious and **healthy snacks** every day. Take baby steps. Your body will begin to experience alkalinity, so you will be less tempted to go back to unhealthy, acid-forming processed foods.

Most of us like snacking. Snacking is not necessarily a bad thing as long as you snack on healthy and nutritious foods. I love preparing my Tupperware with sliced radish, cucumber and carrots! Many of my friends were rather surprised to see me always snacking on fresh vegetables, but eventually they started doing the same thing.

MY OBSERVATION: The more alkaline you go, the more your taste buds will change. Yes! If I was to have some processed sweets or cookies now, I think I would get a headache and nausea. I would not be able to drink a can of Coke, either. At the same time, fresh, organic carrots give my taste buds a nice sensation of something sweet.

Is too much fruit good for you?

Before I discovered the alkaline diet, I thought that all fruits were good for me, even though I felt bloated very often after eating them (I would eat them in excess amounts). I wanted to get healthy, so I decided to eat more fruits. After all, fruits are healthy!

This is certainly true (fruits are healthy), but if we want to do it the alkaline way, we need to know which fruits alkaline-forming and which fruits acid-forming are slightly. Thanks to the alkaline diet, I realized that I should eat some fruits in moderation because they just did not agree with me or my stomach. Choosing more alkaline-forming fruits helped me in my weight loss efforts. I also learned how to eat fruits (more about this later) to achieve the best health results and great energy without experiencing bloating and other digestive issues.

According to research conducted by Dr. Young, who is considered to be the pioneer of the Alkaline Diet, these fruits are alkaline because they have an alkalizing effect on your body once digested and metabolized. What makes them alkaline is their super high mineral content and very low sugar content. If you want to lose weight, you might want to incorporate these into your diet:

- Avocado
- Tomato
- Lemon
- Lime
- Grapefruit
- Fresh Coconut
- Pomegranate
- Watermelon

They are all great in smoothies!

Yes, I was also surprised when I found out that a tomato is a fruit! The definition is simple: scientifically speaking, it is a fruit; however, many cooks refer to it as a vegetable. No matter what you call it, it is extremely alkalizing. Personally, I love making tomato juice with herbs as my aperitif. I make sure I alkalinize my body even before my healthy meal.

Now, let's talk about other fruits. Don't get me wrong, they are not unhealthy or bad for you, it's just that they are not super-alkaline. In general, most fruits (like the fruits listed below) are considered acid-forming because of their high amount of sugar, which is why many alkaline experts recommend reducing the following fruits in your diet.

They are OK in small amounts, it's not that you have to eliminate them all from your diet!

These fruits are moderately acid-forming or neutral:

- Bananas
- Apples
- Apricots
- Currants
- Dates
- Grapes

- Mangos
- Peaches
- Pears
- Prunes
- Raisins
- Raspberries
- Strawberries
- Tropical fruits
- Cantaloupe
- Cranberries
- Honeydew Melon
- Oranges
- Pineapples
- Plums

Meat, caffeine, artificial sweeteners, and fermented foods are highly acid-forming, so that you have a comparison. Fruit is much better for you!

These fruits are more recommended to constitute the 'non-alkaline' 20%-30% of your diet. I also encourage you to use your own instinct and listen to your body. Don't get too obsessed about fruits, there is no need to eliminate them. Just focus on non-sugary fruits as much as you can and use other (moderately acid-forming) fruits as a natural way to satisfy your sweet tooth. Remember to eat fruit between your meals, as a snack, or use them to make a delicious smoothie. Don't juice fruits that are rich in sugar, have them whole or blend them to make a smoothie (with all its natural fiber).

Don't eat fruits as dessert after a meal. Doing this may cause bloating and digestive issues and is not recommended for weight loss efforts.

After learning that some fruits are alkalizing and others are acidifying, I was able to move my diet in a healthier direction. Even though I thought I was already healthy, I learned that some fruits, in exaggerated amounts, disagreed with me and my stomach. My tip for you is to follow your instinct. Take note of which fruits you eat and how your body feels afterwards. Personally, I have noticed that I am naturally attracted to most of the alkaline fruits mentioned above.

Of course, when it comes to fruits, even the most acid-forming fruit is much better for you than processed sweets or fast food. Those are much more acid-forming than slightly acidifying fruits. This is why you shouldn't worry much about fruits. Of course, if you want to lose weight, don't go overboard and make sure that you choose fruits that are more alkaline.

If, for example, you have a choice between a banana and processed chocolate croissants, a banana would be a better choice, obviously. Personally, I like bananas as quick energy boosters, and I always have some around. I love bananas after, or even during, my strenuous workouts. They're the best natural sweets for me ever!

I always choose seasonal, local, and organic fruits. Remember though, fruits are a great tool to help you transition. However, ideally, you want to move more towards vegetables and alkalizing fruits. Treat non-alkaline fruits as a natural raw food treat. You can also add some fruits, like bananas, to your green smoothies to taste. My classic smoothie is spinach, almond milk, and a few slices of banana or dates. It tastes delicious, and it helps me add more alkaline greens into my diet.

Alkaline Ash-Producing Foods

To get started on the alkaline diet, here are the top alkaline ash-producing foods that you can start to include in your diet right now:

Almond, Almond Milk

Almonds, in any type of diet or list, are consistently at the top of the healthiest foods to include. It's also a top alkaline food and is very versatile. You can toast it and add it to salads, smoothies or baked products. You can use it for almond-crusted meats, fish or poultry to balance the pH of a dish. Almonds are also perfect as simple, hassle-free snacks. Just limit the consumption to not more than a handful a day.

Aside from its alkaline effect, almonds also promote other health benefits. These are linked to better lean muscle gain, aids in fat loss (resulting in healthier weight loss) and helps in decreasing levels of cholesterol in the body.

Almond milk is a great alternative to dairy milk. This is healthier and less likely to cause any digestive concerns that regular dairy milk does in sensitive people. It is a great alternative for those who are struggling with weight issues and allergic or intolerance conditions. Just use it in place of milk, such as in smoothies.

Nutritional profile (per 100 grams):

Calcium content: 27%

Protein content: 44%

Iron content: 25%

Artichokes

These are commonly added to salads or in dips, but this humble artichoke can be used as a main ingredient instead of just an addition. Its alkalizing effect helps in raising the pH in the body and in promoting better health. Aside from that, artichokes contain lots of antioxidants that aid in detoxifying the liver and in improving the digestive process.

Artichokes are often seen on top of salads, or used in a dip, but there are a number of reasons why you can bring them to the forefront of your diet. One of those reasons is their alkalinity, helping to raise your body's pH levels. They're also full of antioxidants, help to purify the liver, and aid in digestion.

Use artichokes more often and in larger amounts. For example, grilled artichokes make great pairings with meats to balance the pH.

Nutritional profile (per 100 grams):

Vitamin K: 12%

Vitamin C: 20%

Folates: 17%

Arugula

Calcium is usually abundant in dairy foods, but there are other rich, non-dairy sources as well such as arugula. This is another great leafy green worth knowing and adding to daily meals. This leafy green is more commonly added to detoxifying diet plans. It is one of the top alkaline foods to try. Arugula is abundant in Vitamin A and has impressive calcium content.

Aside from being low in calories, it's also low in cholesterol and fat—which most health-conscious people don't want in their diets, too. On the other hand, it is high in potassium, Vitamins C, K, and A, fiber, and other important nutrients. Arugula is also filled with antioxidants that drive toxins away—and kills free radicals that damage the body.

Nutritional profile (per 100 grams):

Calcium: 16%

Iron: 8%

Vitamin A: 47%

Asparagus

This is an effective food when it comes to promoting alkalinity in the body. This is among the top ranked foods in the alkaline diet, but aside from alkalizing the body, arugula brings so much more. It is known as one of the most traditional detoxifying foods because it's able to act as a diuretic that drives toxins away and speeds up metabolism in the body. It also contains important vitamins and minerals, such as protein, copper, iron, folate, and Vitamins B6, K, E, C, and A, among others.

It is chock full of antioxidants and nutrients. It also has lots of detoxifying properties that promote better health. This crunchy green is also reported to have effective anti-aging effects.

Nutritional profile (per 100 grams):

Vitamin C: 9%

Vitamin A: 15%

Iron: 12%

Avocado & Avocado Oil

Avocado is rich in healthy fats that promote various health benefits. This is also among the top alkaline foods that you should include in daily meals. There are so many ways to add avocados. Try them as part of power-packed smoothies, as sweet addition to salads, as desserts on their own or as dip (guacamole). Avocados are also packed with Vitamin K that promotes alkalinity and other health benefits.

Avocado oil is another powerful alkalizing food. It makes a great substitute to unhealthy acidic oils.

Nutritional profile (per 100 grams):

Vitamin A: 3%

Fiber: 27%

Vitamin C: 17%

Basil

Not all people realize that spices and herbs have notable effects in their bodies. These are more than just aromatics and flavorings. These also influence the acidity or alkalinity of the body. Basil is one of the best herbs that promote alkalinity. Aside from this, basil contains a good amount of flavonoids that promote health and healing.

Nutritional profile (per 100 grams):

Vitamin A: 175%

Calcium: 18%

Vitamin K: 345%

Buckwheat

This is a rising star among the health food circle. It does not contain wheat, even if the name has the word "wheat" in it. This is fast becoming a widely used healthier alternative to wheat. Noodles made of buckwheat have very similar texture to those made of wheat. This makes it a great alternative to wheat pasta, allowing people to enjoy pasta dishes without the negative effects from wheat.

Buckwheat also lowers the acidity in the body, so people do not have to worry about acidity. Aside from its alkaline effects, buckwheat is also a great source of healthy proteins, with a good amount of iron as well. There are so any recipes to try using buckwheat so start adding this to daily meals.

Nutritional profile (per 100 grams):

Protein: 13.3 grams

Calcium: 2%

Iron: 12%

Carrot

These are great vegetables for improved eye health. It also has great alkalizing effects in the body. These are tasty whether raw or cooked. Carrots are rich in carotenoids, vitamins, potassium and fiber.

Nutritional profile (per 100 grams):

Vitamin A: 336%

Calcium: 3%

Vitamin C: 10%

Cauliflower

This belongs to the same vegetable family as Brussels sprouts and broccoli. These are all cruciferous vegetables. These share the same nutritional characteristics and all promote alkaline environments in the body. Cauliflower is a great source of folate. It's also filled with lots of Vitamin C and phytonutrients that help you lose weight and prevent the formation of cancer. It's also a good rice substitute and is one of the most important superfoods around.

Cauliflower, in particular, has a good amount of fiber. This is also a great source of vitamin C, comparable to the amounts found in fruits. Cauliflower is best eaten raw to retain most of its alkaline-promoting compounds.

Nutritional profile (per 100 grams):

Vitamin C: 77%

Iron: 2%

Calcium: 2%

Celery

Some people may not be keen on the taste of raw celery sticks but its nutritional offers are so much worth it. It is a highly alkaline food that can promote balance in the body's pH levels. Celery contains low amounts of calories but it is very filling. This is perfect for those who want to promote alkalinity in the body and those who are trying to lose weight. Munch on fresh celery sticks or add them to smoothies for some more spiciness.

Nutritional profile (per 100 grams):

Vitamin A: 4%

Calcium: 2%

Vitamin C: 2%

Other Alkalizing Foods

Apart from these top alkalizing foods, here are a few more items to add to improve the pH balance in the body.

Alkalizing Protein

Meats and other animal protein sources are top acidifying foods, but this does not mean that you should eliminate protein from your diet. Protein is important in promoting health and wellness. There are protein sources that have alkalizing effect in the body, so make sure to add these:

- Chestnuts

- Almonds

- Millet

- Tofu (fermented)

- Tempeh (fermented)

- Whey Protein Powder

Alkalizing Sweeteners

Sugar is an acidifying food ingredient. Natural sugars in food have alkalizing effect but added ones like added refined sugars will acidify the body. Artificial sweeteners used in place of refined white sugar are also acidifying. One safe, alkalizing artificial sweetener is Stevia.

Alkalizing Spices & Seasonings

Seasonings and spices are simple and easy ways to turn acidic meals to more alkaline.

- Herbs (all)

- Cinnamon

- Chili Pepper

- Curry

- Ginger

- Miso

- Sea Salt

- Mustard

- Tamari

Other Alkalizing Foods

A few more other foods that can help in reversing acidity and restoring pH balance in the body include:

- Alkaline Antioxidant Water

- Mineral Water

- Bee Pollen

- Apple Cider Vinegar

- Green Juices

- Fresh Fruit Juice

- Molasses, blackstrap

- Soured Dairy Products

- Probiotic Cultures

- Veggie Juices

- Lecithin Granules

Alkalizing Minerals

Minerals in food and supplements can also help in alkalizing the body. The best ones are:

- Sodium: pH 14

- Potassium: pH 14

- Cesium: pH 14

- Calcium: pH 12

- Magnesium: pH 9

Alkaline Recipe Box:

Breakfast Recipes

Easy Pumpkin Patties

Total Time: 20 minutes
Serves: 4 Servings

Ingredients:

2 eggs

6 cups pumpkin, grated

1/2 cup alkaline breadcrumbs

Olive oil

1 tsp ground cumin seeds

1/2 cup plain flour

2 onion, chopped

1/4 cup coriander, chopped

Pepper

Salt

Directions:

1. Add all ingredients in mixing bowl except breadcrumbs and oil. Mix well until combined.

2. Make patties from mixture and roll in breadcrumbs. Place patties in refrigerator for 30 minutes.

3. Add some olive oil in pan over medium heat.

4. Remove patties from refrigerator and fry on pan for about 4 minutes each side until golden brown.

5. Serve hot and enjoy.

Nutrition Facts

Servings: 4

Amount per serving

Calories	**293**

	% Daily Value*
Total Fat 4.5g	6%
Saturated Fat 1.4g	7%
Cholesterol 82mg	27%
Sodium 191mg	8%
Total Carbohydrate 57g	21%
Dietary Fiber 12.9g	46%
Total Sugars 15.5g	
Protein 11g	
Vitamin D 8mcg	39%
Calcium 153mg	12%
Iron 7mg	41%
Potassium 916mg	19%

Delicious Halloumi and Carrot Patties

Total Time: 25 minutes
Serves: 3 Servings

Ingredients:

1 egg white

2 tbsp fennel seed

2 tbsp rice flour

1 onion, grated

1 garlic clove, minced

4 oz halloumi, grated

1 lemon juice

2 tbsp coriander

4 spring onions

4 large carrots, grated

Olive oil

Directions:

1. Add 2 tablespoon of olive oil in pan over medium heat then add fennel seed and sauté for 3 minutes. Turn off the heat and set aside.

2. Mix all ingredients into the bowl with fennel seed and olive oil.

3. Take handful of mixture and make small patties and sear till golden on each side.

4. Place patties in pre-heated oven at 175 F for 15 minutes.

Nutrition Facts

Servings: 3

Amount per serving

Calories	108

	% Daily Value*
Total Fat 1.1g	1%
Saturated Fat 0.1g	1%
Cholesterol 0mg	0%
Sodium 86mg	4%
Total Carbohydrate 22.1g	8%
Dietary Fiber 5.4g	19%
Total Sugars 6.9g	
Protein 3.8g	
Vitamin D 0mcg	0%
Calcium 104mg	8%
Iron 1mg	8%
Potassium 512mg	11%

Coconut Chia Strawberry Pudding

Total Time: 20 minutes
Serves: 4 Servings

Ingredients:

4 tbsp chia seeds

3/4 cup milk

1 tsp vanilla extract

3 tbsp maple syrup

11/4 cups plain yogurt

Coconut chips, toasted

6 oz strawberries

1/4 tsp salt

Directions:

1.   In a mixing bowl add chia seeds, vanilla extract, salt, maple syrup, plain yogurt and milk. Whisk well until blended.

2.   Add strawberries in blender and blend until purred.

3.   Add strawberry puree into the chia mixture and mix well.

4.   Cover the mixture and refrigerate for 2 hours.

5. After 2 hours spoon the pudding into four bowls and top with coconut chips.

6. Serve immediately and enjoy.

Nutrition Facts

Servings: 4

Amount per serving

Calories	241

	% Daily Value*
Total Fat 5.7g	7%
Saturated Fat 4.8g	24%
Cholesterol 14mg	5%
Sodium 330mg	14%
Total Carbohydrate 31.9g	12%
Dietary Fiber 1.7g	6%
Total Sugars 27.8g	
Protein 11.7g	
Vitamin D 0mcg	1%
Calcium 381mg	29%
Iron 1mg	4%
Potassium 519mg	11%

Simple Tofu Scramble

Total Time: 30 minutes
Serves: 3 Servings

Ingredients:

1 block extra firm tofu, crumbled

1/2 tsp turmeric powder

1 tsp cumin powder

1 tsp garlic powder

1 small onion, diced

1/4 cup cauliflower, diced

1 zucchini, diced

1 bell pepper, chopped

1 tsp oil

Pepper

Salt

Directions:

1.   Add oil in large pan over medium heat once oil is hot then add onion and sauté for 5 minutes.

2. Add crumbled tofu and seasoning in pan and cook for another 5 minutes. Season with pepper and salt to taste.

3. Add diced veggies in pan and cook for 10 minutes.

4. Serve warm with tortillas and enjoy.

Nutrition Facts

Servings: 3

Amount per serving

Calories	**55**

	% Daily Value*
Total Fat 2g	3%
Saturated Fat 0.2g	1%
Cholesterol 0mg	0%
Sodium 63mg	3%
Total Carbohydrate 9.1g	3%
Dietary Fiber 2.2g	8%
Total Sugars 4.6g	
Protein 2g	
Vitamin D 0mcg	0%
Calcium 29mg	2%
Iron 1mg	6%
Potassium 338mg	7%

Healthy Quinoa and Apple Breakfast

Total Time: 30 minutes
Serves: 4 Servings

Ingredients:

1 cup quinoa

3 cups water

3 tsp cinnamon

3 large apples, peeled and core

1 tbsp honey

Directions:

1. Chop apples into the small pieces.

2. Add chopped apples, quinoa and water into the saucepan. Bring to boil.

3. Cover saucepan with lid and simmer for 25 minutes or until apples will be soften and quinoa absorb the water.

4. Add cinnamon and stir well. Transfer mixture into the four serving bowls.

5. Drizzle with honey and serve.

Nutrition Facts

Servings: 4

Amount per serving

Nutrition Facts

Servings: 4

| **Calories** | **264** |

	% Daily Value*
Total Fat 2.9g	**4%**
Saturated Fat 0.3g	**2%**
Cholesterol 0mg	**0%**
Sodium 9mg	**0%**
Total Carbohydrate 56.1g	**20%**
Dietary Fiber 8g	**28%**
Total Sugars 21.8g	
Protein 6.5g	
Vitamin D 0mcg	0%
Calcium 44mg	3%
Iron 3mg	16%
Potassium 430mg	9%

Healthy Avocado Breakfast Salad

Total Time: 15 minutes
Serves: 4 Servings

Ingredients:

2 avocados, diced

2 tbsp lemon juice

2 tbsp extra virgin olive oil

1 small onion, sliced

1 cucumber, sliced

1 lb roma tomatoes

1/4 cup cilantro, chopped

1/8 tsp black pepper

1 tsp sea salt

Directions:

1. Add onion, avocado, cucumber, tomatoes and cilantro into the mixing bowl. Mix well.

2. Drizzle with lemon juice and olive oil. Toss well to combine.

3. Just before serving add black pepper and salt.

4. Serve immediately and enjoy.

Nutrition Facts

Servings: 4

Amount per serving

Calories	**306**

	% Daily Value*
Total Fat 27g	35%
Saturated Fat 5.2g	26%
Cholesterol 0mg	0%
Sodium 484mg	21%
Total Carbohydrate 17.7g	6%
Dietary Fiber 8.9g	32%
Total Sugars 5.7g	
Protein 3.7g	
Vitamin D 0mcg	0%
Calcium 41mg	3%
Iron 1mg	7%
Potassium 908mg	19%

Lunch Recipes

Easy Chickpea and Kale Mash

Total Time: 20 minutes
Serves: 2 Servings

Ingredients:

14 oz fresh chickpeas, cooked

3 tbsp garlic, chopped

1 bunch kale, rinsed and drained

1/2 tsp thyme, dried

2 tbsp extra virgin olive oil

2 tbsp liquid aminos

1 shallot, chopped

Sea salt

Directions:

1.   In pan heat olive oil over medium heat once oil is hot then add garlic and shallot, sauté for 5 minutes until soften.

2.   Add drained kale and stir well and cook until kale is wilted.

3. Now add chickpeas and cook about 6 minutes then add remaining ingredients and stir.

4. Finally using masher mashed the chickpeas and serve.

Nutrition Facts

Servings: 4

Amount per serving

Calories	**154**
	% Daily Value*
Total Fat 7.9g	10%
Saturated Fat 1.1g	6%
Cholesterol 0mg	0%
Sodium 514mg	22%
Total Carbohydrate 17.8g	6%
Dietary Fiber 3.7g	13%
Total Sugars 1.6g	
Protein 5.9g	
Vitamin D 0mcg	0%
Calcium 119mg	9%
Iron 2mg	12%
Potassium 479mg	10%

Quinoa and Kale Salad

Total Time: 20 minutes
Serves: 4 Servings

Ingredients:

1/2 quinoa, cooked

4 cups kale, chopped

1 lemon zest

3 tbsp fresh lemon juice

4 tbsp olive oil

4 tbsp apple cider vinegar

1/2 cup almonds, sliced

1/2 cup pomegranate seeds

1 avocado, diced

2 tbsp pecans, chopped

Black pepper

1 tsp sea salt

Directions:

1.   In small bowl, whisk together lemon zest, lemon juice, apple cider vinegar and olive oil. Set aside.

2.   In large mixing bowl, add kale, quinoa, avocado, pecans and pomegranate. Mix well.

3.   Pour dressing on top of salad and toss well to combine.

4.   Season with pepper and salt to taste.

5.   Serve immediately and enjoy.

Nutrition Facts

Servings: 4

Amount per serving

Calories	333

	% Daily Value*
Total Fat 30g	39%
Saturated Fat 4.6g	23%
Cholesterol 0mg	0%
Sodium 503mg	22%
Total Carbohydrate 14.5g	5%
Dietary Fiber 6g	21%
Total Sugars 1.1g	
Protein 5.6g	
Vitamin D 0mcg	0%
Calcium 130mg	10%
Iron 2mg	10%
Potassium 688mg	15%

Delicious Cauliflower Tabouli

Total Time: 15 minutes
Serves: 4 Servings

Ingredients:

1/2 head of cauliflower, cut into florets

1 cucumber, peeled and diced

1 bunch green onions, chopped

2 cups tomatoes, diced

3 bunch parsley, chopped

2 tbsp fresh mint, chopped

3 tbsp fresh lemon juice

1/3 cup extra virgin olive oil

1/4 tsp ground black pepper

1/2 tsp sea salt

Directions:

1. Place cauliflower florets into the food processor. Pulse until get couscous consistency.

2. Transfer cauliflower mixture into the large mixing bowl.

3. Add cucumber, green onion, tomatoes, parsley, mint, lemon juice and olive oil. Toss well to combine.

4. Season with pepper and salt to taste.

5. Serve immediately and enjoy.

Nutrition Facts

Servings: 4

Amount per serving

Calories	184
	% Daily Value*
Total Fat 17.2g	22%
Saturated Fat 2.6g	13%
Cholesterol 0mg	0%
Sodium 253mg	11%
Total Carbohydrate 8.6g	3%
Dietary Fiber 2.6g	9%
Total Sugars 4.7g	
Protein 2.1g	
Vitamin D 0mcg	0%
Calcium 36mg	3%
Iron 1mg	6%
Potassium 455mg	10%

Spicy Honey Tofu

Total Time: 20 minutes
Serves: 4 Servings

Ingredients:

14 oz extra firm tofu, cut into cubes

1 tbsp olive oil

2 tsp sesame seeds

1/2 tsp basil, dried

1/4 tsp cayenne powder

1 tsp apple cider vinegar

1 1/2 tbsp honey

2 tbsp sriracha chili sauce

1 tsp Worcestershire sauce

1 tbsp soy sauce

1 green Chile, chopped

1 inch ginger, chopped

3 garlic cloves, chopped

Black pepper

Garlic salt

Directions:

1. Heat olive oil in non-stick pan over medium heat once oil is hot add garlic, green Chile and ginger sauté for 3 minutes.

2. Now add tofu and sprinkle some garlic salt to taste, sauté it for 8 minutes or until golden brown.

3. In small bowl add honey, soy sauce, cayenne powder, sriracha chili sauce and Worcestershire sauce. Mix well.

4. Add honey mixture into the tofu and mix well until well coated. Cook for 2 minutes.

5. Add sesame seeds and basil leaves. Mix well.

6. Serve hot and enjoy.

Nutrition Facts

Servings: 4

Amount per serving

Calories	141

	% Daily Value*
Total Fat 8.4g	11%
Saturated Fat 1.5g	7%
Cholesterol 0mg	0%
Sodium 260mg	11%
Total Carbohydrate 10.3g	4%
Dietary Fiber 1.3g	5%
Total Sugars 7.5g	
Protein 8.9g	

Nutrition Facts

Servings: 4

Vitamin D 0mcg	0%
Calcium 220mg	17%
Iron 2mg	11%
Potassium 186mg	4%

Spicy and Tasty Tuna Salad

Total Time: 10 minutes
Serves: 2 Servings

Ingredients:

2 cans tuna, drained

1/4 tsp red pepper flakes

1/4 tsp dill

1/4 tsp black pepper

1 cup carrot, shredded

4 celery stalks, chopped

1/8 cup sriracha sauce

1/8 cup mustard

1/2 cup plain yogurt

Directions:

1. Add all ingredients into large mixing bowl and mix well until combine.

2. Serve immediately and enjoy.

Nutrition Facts

Servings: 4

Amount per serving

Calories	**201**

	% Daily Value*
Total Fat 7.6g	**10%**
Saturated Fat 1.8g	**9%**
Cholesterol 29mg	**10%**
Sodium 98mg	**4%**
Total Carbohydrate 5.4g	**2%**
Dietary Fiber 1g	**3%**
Total Sugars 3.7g	
Protein 25.7g	
Vitamin D 0mcg	0%
Calcium 75mg	6%
Iron 1mg	4%
Potassium 500mg	

Sweet potato and Zucchini Fritters

Total Time: 25 minutes

Serves: 12 Servings

Ingredients:

3 eggs

3 cups zucchini, grated

3 tbsp coconut oil

2 spring onion, sliced

1 1/4 cups sweet potato, peeled and grated

1 tbsp coriander, chopped

1 tbsp parsley, chopped

2/3 cup almond meal

1/4 tsp sea salt

Directions:

1.   Add grated sweet potato and zucchini in colander with sea salt and set aside for 15 minutes.

2.   After 15 minutes squeeze out excess moisture.

3.   Add zucchini and sweet potato mixture in large mixing bowl with remaining ingredients except coconut oil. Mix well.

4.   Heat coconut oil in frying pan over medium heat. Using spoon scoop out fritter mixture and place in the pan and flatten a little.

5. Cook fritter until edges golden brown.

6. Serve hot and enjoy.

Nutrition Facts

Servings: 4

Amount per serving

Calories	**299**

	% Daily Value*
Total Fat 21.7g	**28%**
Saturated Fat 10.5g	**52%**
Cholesterol 123mg	**41%**
Sodium 196mg	**9%**
Total Carbohydrate 20g	**7%**
Dietary Fiber 5.2g	**19%**
Total Sugars 6.6g	
Protein 9.9g	
Vitamin D 12mcg	58%
Calcium 80mg	6%
Iron 4mg	21%
Potassium 700mg	15%

Quick and Simple Egg and Avocado Salad

Total Time: 10 minutes
Serves: 4 Servings

Ingredients:

1 avocado, ripe and slightly mashed

8 eggs, boiled and chopped

1/2 tsp sea salt

2 tbsp fresh lemon juice

Directions:

1.   In a mixing bowl combine together avocado, eggs, sea salt and lemon juice.

2.   Toss well until combine.

3.   Serve immediately and enjoy.

Nutrition Facts

Servings: 4

Amount per serving

Calories	230
	% Daily Value*
Total Fat 18.6g	**24%**
Saturated Fat 4.9g	**24%**

Nutrition Facts

Servings: 4

Cholesterol 327mg	**109%**
Sodium 362mg	**16%**
Total Carbohydrate 5.2g	**2%**
Dietary Fiber 3.4g	**12%**
Total Sugars 1.1g	
Protein 12.1g	
Vitamin D 31mcg	154%
Calcium 53mg	4%
Iron 2mg	11%
Potassium 371mg	8%

<u>Dinner Recipes</u>

Roasted Vegetable Pasta

Total Time: 50 minutes
Serves: 4 Servings

Ingredients:

2 eggs

8 oz organic wholegrain pasta

8 oz mushrooms, quartered

1 tbsp parsley, chopped

1/4 cup parmesan, grated

1 garlic clove, chopped

4 oz bacon, cut into 1 inch pieces

1 tbsp olive oil

1 small cauliflower head, cut into florets

Pepper

Salt

Directions:

1. Preheat the oven at 400 F.

2. In bowl, add cauliflower, mushroom, pepper, salt and oil. Toss well and place on baking tray.

3. Roast mushroom and cauliflower in preheated oven for 25 minutes.

4. Cook pasta according to the packet directions.

5. Cook bacon in pan pour off tbsp of the grease from pan, add garlic in pan and cook for 30 second. Turn off heat.

6. In bowl, mix together parsley, cheese, egg, pepper and salt.

7. Drain pasta and mix with egg mixture and cauliflower and mushroom mixture into the pan with bacon.

8. Cook in pan for 10 minutes and serve hot.

Nutrition Facts

Servings: 4

Amount per serving

Calories	393

	% Daily Value*
Total Fat 19.1g	24%
Saturated Fat 5.3g	27%
Cholesterol 155mg	52%
Sodium 746mg	32%
Total Carbohydrate 33.8g	12%
Dietary Fiber 0.6g	2%
Total Sugars 1.2g	

Nutrition Facts

Servings: 4

Protein 21.6g

Vitamin D 212mcg	1059%
Calcium 28mg	2%
Iron 4mg	25%
Potassium 481mg	10%

Yummy Egg Stuffed Cucumber

Total Time: 15 minutes
Serves: 4 Servings

Ingredients:

1 large cucumber, 12 inches

4 hardboiled eggs, peeled

1/4 tsp ground pepper

2 tsp Dijon mustard

2 tbsp chopped parsley

1 celery stalk, diced

1/4 cup plain yogurt

Pinch of cayenne pepper

1/8 teaspoon salt

Directions:

1. In a mixing bowl, mash eggs with back of fork. Stir in parsley, celery, yogurt, mustard, pepper and salt.

2. Cut cucumber in half then cut each piece in half lengthwise.

3. Scoop out cucumber seeds.

4. Divide the eggs mixture into the 4 equal portions and stuffed in four cucumber boats.

5. Sprinkle cayenne pepper over the top of each boat.

6. Serve immediately and enjoy.

Nutrition Facts

Servings: 4

Amount per serving

Calories	89

	% Daily Value*
Total Fat 4.8g	6%
Saturated Fat 1.6g	8%
Cholesterol 165mg	55%
Sodium 180mg	8%
Total Carbohydrate 4.6g	2%
Dietary Fiber 0.6g	2%
Total Sugars 2.8g	
Protein 7.1g	

Nutrition Facts

Servings: 4

Vitamin D 15mcg	77%
Calcium 70mg	5%
Iron 1mg	7%
Potassium 233mg	5%

Delicious Marinated Eggplant

Total Time: 2 hours
Serves: 4 Servings

Ingredients:

18 oz eggplant, cut into slices

1 bell pepper, roasted and diced

3/4 cup olive oil, divided

1 tbsp parsley, chopped

1 garlic clove, minced

1 small jalapeno pepper, seeded and chopped

1/4 tsp pepper

1 tsp salt

Directions:

1. Place eggplant slices in plate and sprinkle with salt both the side. Brush the eggplant with oil. Set aside for 30 minutes.

2. In a pan, heat olive oil over the medium-high heat and place eggplant onto the pan cook both the side until golden brown.

3. Transfer the eggplant slices in bowl and add bell pepper, parsley, garlic, jalapeno, pepper and salt in bowl toss well until combined.

4. Cover the bowl with lid and marinate in refrigerator for 1 hour.

Nutrition Facts

Servings: 4

Amount per serving

Calories	367

	% Daily Value*
Total Fat 38.1g	49%
Saturated Fat 5.4g	27%
Cholesterol 0mg	0%
Sodium 585mg	25%
Total Carbohydrate 10.2g	4%
Dietary Fiber 5g	18%
Total Sugars 5.4g	
Protein 1.6g	
Vitamin D 0mcg	0%
Calcium 18mg	1%
Iron 1mg	3%
Potassium 359mg	8%

Crispy Tofu Steaks

Total Time: 30 minutes
Serves: 4 Servings

Ingredients:

1 egg

14 oz firm tofu, drained and sliced 1 inch thick

1 cup alkaline breadcrumbs (look for gluten free)

1/3 cup coconut oil

1 tbsp white vinegar

3 tbsp scallion, minced

3 tbsp ginger, minced

Salt

Directions:

1. In small bowl, combine together ginger, salt, vinegar, scallion and 1/3 cup oil.

2. Beat the egg in another bowl and set aside.

3. In shallow dish add breadcrumbs.

4. Heat remaining oil in pan over medium heat.

5.   Dip tofu slices in egg then coat with breadcrumbs and fry on hot pan until golden brown and crispy. About 8 minutes.

6.   Serve hot tofu slices with ginger mixture and enjoy.

Nutrition Facts

Servings: 4

Amount per serving

Calories	**348**

	% Daily Value*
Total Fat 24.8g	32%
Saturated Fat 17.2g	86%
Cholesterol 41mg	14%
Sodium 225mg	10%
Total Carbohydrate 21.2g	8%
Dietary Fiber 2.1g	8%
Total Sugars 2.4g	
Protein 13.1g	
Vitamin D 4mcg	19%
Calcium 255mg	20%
Iron 3mg	17%
Potassium 215mg	5%

Healthy Sautéed Leeks and Cabbage

Total Time: 20 minutes
Serves: 2 Servings

Ingredients:

1 leek, chopped

2 tbsp soy sauce

1/2 green cabbage, sliced

1 tbsp rice wine vinegar

1/2 tsp ginger, minced

2 garlic cloves, minced

3 bacon slices, diced

Directions:

1. Sauté bacon until crispy then removes from pan and crushed with spoon.

2. Add leek in pan and sauté for 4 minutes over medium heat.

3. Add ginger and garlic and cook for another 1 minute.

4. Add soy sauce, vinegar and crushed bacon in pan. Stir well.

5. Add cabbage and cook for 7 minutes.

6. Serve warm and enjoy.

Nutrition Facts

Servings: 2

Amount per serving

Calories	**50**

	% Daily Value*
Total Fat 0.4g	1%
Saturated Fat 0.1g	1%
Cholesterol 1mg	0%
Sodium 923mg	40%
Total Carbohydrate 8.9g	3%
Dietary Fiber 1.1g	4%
Total Sugars 2.1g	
Protein 2.1g	
Vitamin D 0mcg	0%
Calcium 36mg	3%
Iron 1mg	8%
Potassium 137mg	3%

Salmon with Mushroom and Spinach

Total Time: 35 minutes
Serves: 2 Servings

Ingredients:

1 lb salmon fillets, with skin

1 tbsp lemon juice

3 tbsp olive oil

1/2 tsp garlic powder

1 cup tomato, chopped

2 cups fresh spinach, chopped

2 medium mushrooms, sliced

2 oz Parmesan cheese, grated

Black pepper

Salt

Directions:

1. Preheat the oven at 375 F.

2. Wash salmon fillet and dry with paper towel.

3. Season with pepper and salt.

4. Spray baking dish with cooking spray and place salmon fillet skin side down in dish.

5. Combine remaining ingredients except parmesan cheese and spoon over the fish fillet.

6. Bake in preheated oven for 25 minutes.

7. Sprinkle grated parmesan cheese and serve.

Nutrition Facts

Servings: 4

Amount per serving

Calories   301

                                                      % Daily Value*

Total Fat 20.7g   **27%**

  Saturated Fat 4.6g   **23%**

Cholesterol 60mg   **20%**

Sodium 195mg   **8%**

Total Carbohydrate 3.4g   **1%**

  Dietary Fiber 1g   **4%**

  Total Sugars 1.6g

Protein 27.7g

Vitamin D 32mcg   162%

Calcium 185mg   14%

Iron 2mg   8%

Potassium 663mg   14%

Tasty Veggie Quinoa Patties

Total Time: 20 minutes
Serves: 8 Servings

Ingredients:

3 cup quinoa, cooked

3 eggs

2 tbsp olive oil

2 cups alkaline breadcrumbs

1/2 parmesan cheese, grated

1 cup spinach, chopped

4 green onions, diced

1 carrot, shredded

2 garlic cloves

2 tbsp parsley, chopped

1/2 tsp Salt

Directions:

1. Combine all ingredients except oil in bowl mix well until all combined.

2. Let the mixture rest for 10 minutes.

3. Heat the oil in large pan over medium heat.

4. Form the mixture into small round patties and cook patties in pan for 2 minutes.

5. Flip the patties and cook for 2 minutes until both sides are golden brown.

6. Let cool for 5 minutes before serving.

7. Serve with sauce and enjoy.

Nutrition Facts

Servings: 8

Amount per serving

Calories   403

	% Daily Value*
Total Fat 10.5g	13%
Saturated Fat 1.8g	9%
Cholesterol 61mg	20%
Sodium 383mg	17%
Total Carbohydrate 62.2g	23%
Dietary Fiber 6.2g	22%
Total Sugars 2.4g	
Protein 15.1g	
Vitamin D 6mcg	29%
Calcium 104mg	8%
Iron 5mg	27%
Potassium 508mg	11%

Simple Lemon Wild Salmon

Total Time: 25 minutes
Serves: 4 Servings

Ingredients:

1 lb wild salmon

1/2 tsp parsley

1/2 tsp tarragon

2 tbsp lemon juice

1/2 tsp dill weeds

3 garlic cloves, minced

1 tbsp olive oil

Directions:

1. Preheat the oven at 300 F.

2. Add olive oil, minced garlic, lemon juice and herbs in bowl and mix well.

3. Spray baking sheet with cooking spray then place salmon on baking sheet and spared herbs mixture over the salmon.

4. Bake salmon about 20 minutes.

5. Serve salmon with steam rice and enjoy.

Nutrition Facts	
Servings: 4	
Amount per serving	
Calories	242
	% Daily Value*
Total Fat 12.8g	**16%**
Saturated Fat 2g	**10%**
Cholesterol 81mg	**27%**

Nutrition Facts

Servings: 4

Sodium 66mg		**3%**
Total Carbohydrate 1g		**0%**
Dietary Fiber 0.1g		**0%**
Total Sugars 0.2g		
Protein 29.1g		
Vitamin D 0mcg		0%
Calcium 25mg		2%
Iron 1mg		7%
Potassium 738mg		16%

Crustless Cheese Spinach Quiche

Total Time: 25 minutes
Serves: 6 Servings

Ingredients:

9 oz frozen spinach, chopped

3/4 cup cheddar cheese, shredded

3/4 cup liquid egg substitute

1/4 cup green pepper, chopped

1/4 cup onions, chopped

Directions:

1. Microwave the spinach for 2 minutes on high.

2. Spray muffin dish with cooking spray.

3. Add the egg substitute, peppers, cheese, spinach and onions in bowl.

4. Mix well and divide among the muffin cups.

5. Bake at 350 F for 20 minutes. Serve warm and enjoy.

Nutrition Facts

Servings: 6

Amount per serving

Calories	86

	% Daily Value*
Total Fat 4.9g	6%
Saturated Fat 3g	15%
Cholesterol 15mg	5%
Sodium 182mg	8%
Total Carbohydrate 2.6g	1%
Dietary Fiber 1.1g	4%
Total Sugars 0.7g	
Protein 8.6g	
Vitamin D 2mcg	10%
Calcium 162mg	12%
Iron 2mg	10%
Potassium 312mg	7%

Healthy Tomato and Spinach Frittata

Total Time: 15 minutes
Serves: 4 Servings

Ingredients:

6 eggs

1/2 cup onion, chopped

4 oz fresh baby spinach leaves

1/2 tsp olive oil

2 egg whites

2 tomatoes, chopped

1 tbsp basil leaves, chopped

1/4 tsp black pepper

1/4 tsp salt

Directions:

1. Preheat the oven to 400 F.

2. In a bowl, whisk eggs and egg whites together.

3. Fold egg whites and egg mixture in tomatoes, spinach and onion.

4. Mix in the basil, salt and pepper.

5. Grease, the large non-stick pan with oil and heat the pan over medium heat.

6. Pour the egg mixture into the pan and cook for 1 minute.

7. Transfer pan into the oven and bake for 6 minutes or until golden brown.

8. Remove frittata from oven and let it cool for 5 minutes then cut into wedges and serve.

Nutrition Facts

Servings: 4

Amount per serving

Calories	**132**

	% Daily Value*
Total Fat 7.4g	10%
Saturated Fat 2.2g	11%
Cholesterol 246mg	82%
Sodium 282mg	12%
Total Carbohydrate 5.5g	2%
Dietary Fiber 1.7g	6%
Total Sugars 3g	
Protein 11.6g	
Vitamin D 23mcg	116%
Calcium 76mg	6%
Iron 2mg	13%
Potassium 444mg	9%

Quick Sautéed Shallots with Carrots

Total Time: 20 minutes
Serves: 4 Servings

Ingredients:

1/2 cup shallots

1 lb carrots

1/4 tsp cumin

1 tbsp olive oil

1/2 tsp fresh mint

1 tsp fresh cilantro

1/4 tsp red chili flakes

1/2 tsp fresh parsley

1 tsp salt

Directions:

1. Peel the carrot and cut it into julienne by hand then dice the shallots.

2. Add olive oil in large pan over medium heat.

3. Add shallots and carrots, in pan and sauté 3 minutes. Then add spices and herbs and cook for 3 minutes.

4. Serve warm and enjoy.

Nutrition Facts

Servings: 4

Amount per serving

Calories	92

	% Daily Value*
Total Fat 3.6g	5%
Saturated Fat 0.5g	3%
Cholesterol 0mg	0%
Sodium 809mg	35%
Total Carbohydrate 14.6g	5%
Dietary Fiber 2.8g	10%
Total Sugars 5.6g	
Protein 1.5g	
Vitamin D 0mcg	0%
Calcium 47mg	4%
Iron 1mg	4%
Potassium 434mg	9%

Tasty Tomato and Carrot Soup

Total Time: 1 hour 20 minutes
Serves: 8 Servings

Ingredients:

1 carrot, peeled and cut into small pieces

2 potato, peeled and diced

1 cup coriander, chopped

2 garlic clove, minced

1 tbsp ginger, grated

1 onion, chopped

2 tomatoes, chopped

4 tbsp olive oil

1 tsp pepper

1 tsp cumin

5 cups water

2 tsp salt

Directions:

1. In a saucepan heat olive oil over medium heat.

2. Add onion, ginger, garlic and carrots in pan and sauté for 5 minutes over medium heat.

3. Add tomatoes, potatoes and chopped coriander sauté for further 5 minutes.

4. Add remaining ingredients and bring to boil.

5. Cover pan with lid and simmer over medium-low heat for 60 minutes. Add more water if necessary.

6. Puree soup with blender until completely smooth.

7. Serve hot and enjoy.

Nutrition Facts

Servings: 8

Amount per serving

Calories	112

	% Daily Value*
Total Fat 7.2g	9%
Saturated Fat 1g	5%
Cholesterol 0mg	0%
Sodium 597mg	26%
Total Carbohydrate 11.7g	4%
Dietary Fiber 2.1g	7%
Total Sugars 2.2g	
Protein 1.6g	
Vitamin D 0mcg	0%
Calcium 26mg	2%
Iron 1mg	5%
Potassium 328mg	7%

Quinoa Stuffed Bell Peppers

Total Time: 40 minutes
Serves: 2 Servings

Ingredients:

2 bell peppers, cut into half

1/2 cup quinoa, cooked

1/2 cup goat cheese, crumbled

1 cup cherry tomatoes, quartered

8 oz asparagus, trimmed and cut into 1/4 inch pieces

1/4 tsp olive oil

1 tbsp lemon juice

1 garlic clove, minced

Pepper

Salt

Directions:

1.   Preheat the oven at 400 F. Spray baking tray with non-stick cooking spray.

2.   Place bell peppers on baking tray. Drizzle with olive oil and season with pepper and salt.

3. Place baking tray in oven and bake for 15 minutes. Remove tray from oven and set aside.

4. In a bowl, add cooked quinoa, lemon juice, garlic, olive oil and pepper mix well until combined.

5. Add tomatoes and asparagus in quinoa bowl. Mix well.

6. Stuffed quinoa in bell peppers halves and place crumbled cheese over the top of each pepper.

7. Place stuffed peppers in oven and bake for 5 minutes until cheese is melted.

8. Serve immediately and enjoy.

Nutrition Facts

Servings: 2

Amount per serving

Calories	245
	% Daily Value*
Total Fat 4g	5%
Saturated Fat 0.6g	3%
Cholesterol 1mg	0%
Sodium 93mg	4%
Total Carbohydrate 44.9g	16%
Dietary Fiber 8.1g	29%
Total Sugars 10.7g	
Protein 10.8g	
Vitamin D 0mcg	0%
Calcium 74mg	6%
Iron 5mg	29%

Nutrition Facts

Servings: 2

Potassium 922mg   20%

Yummy Sweet Potato Soup

Total Time: 35 minutes
Serves: 4 Servings

Ingredients:

1 lb sweet potatoes, peeled and diced

3/4 cup cream

2 garlic clove, minced

2 onions, chopped

10 oz carrots, peeled and diced

4 cups vegetable stock

3 tbsp olive oil

Pepper

Salt

Directions:

1.   Heat oven at 200 F.

2.   Place carrots and sweet potatoes onto the roasting tray and drizzle with 2 tbsp olive oil and season with pepper and salt.

3.   Place tray in oven and roast for 25 minutes.

4.   In a sauce pan, add 1 tablespoon olive oil over the medium-high heat.

5.   Add onion in pan sauté for 10 minutes then add garlic and vegetable stock.

6.   Remove roasted vegetables from oven and let it cool for 5 minutes.

7.   Add roasted vegetables in sauce pan and blend it with blender until get smooth mixture. Stir cream.

8.   Serve hot and enjoy.

Nutrition Facts

Servings: 4

Amount per serving

Calories	306
	% Daily Value*
Total Fat 13.3g	17%
Saturated Fat 3.1g	16%
Cholesterol 9mg	3%
Sodium 115mg	5%
Total Carbohydrate 45.7g	17%
Dietary Fiber 7.6g	27%
Total Sugars 7.3g	

Nutrition Facts

Servings: 4

Protein 3.4g

Vitamin D 0mcg	0%
Calcium 69mg	5%
Iron 1mg	6%
Potassium 1255mg	27%

14 Day Alkaline Diet Meal Plan

An alkaline meal plan consists of foods that contain strength, power and endurance. Our bodies require about 20% of acid-forming foods in the diet to function properly.

When these foods are properly digested with alkaline-promoting foods, the acid alkaline balance is achieved and maintained leading to our bodies operating at optimal levels. When the food is properly digested the body absorbs the optimum nutrients. This way we attain optimum performance in whatever we do.

However, if this balance is not achieved or maintained and the acidic-foods are not properly digested, the body develops a condition known as low-grade or chronic acidosis.

Improper combination of foods usually leads to indigestion. Carbohydrates which are made up of starches and sugars ferment while the indigested proteins putrefy. This causes the blood and body tissues to hold the excess acids which have not been digested and as a result, alkaline minerals from bones, muscles and other areas of the body are drained to neutralize the acidity and this compromises our health.

As a result, the cells lose energy and the immune system is compromised making it weaker while health is drained. The immune system is weakened and the acidified cells lose their energy and power to protect our bodies and fight illnesses and diseases naturally. The muscles, tendons, ligaments, joints, organs, cells and bones give in and conditions and diseases plague our lives. We start getting nutrient deficiencies, joint and bone diseases, colon and digestive problems, damage to muscles, tendons and ligaments among other conditions.

Your cells need oxygen and energy to perform all the functions that sustain life whether it is digesting the food you eat, eliminating the toxins or circulating the blood, but the acidity in the cells deprive them of performing these functions. The organs become strained to detoxify the body of the acidity.

An alkaline diet can save our bodies from this state and in fact, they can reverse the acid-forming health conditions. When you adopt an acid alkaline balance diet by eating the required quantity of acid-forming foods and a high amount of alkaline foods, you encourage your body to alkalize the acidity by itself. The body cells are strengthened and they make the immune system strong.

A strong immunity keeps us healthy and helps the body to repair, rejuvenate, regenerate and replenish the nerves, muscles, bones, ligaments and the whole body for optimum physical, mental and athletic performance. The body is able to carry out all the biological performance as it was meant to do. If you want to maintain your natural pH balance, you need to follow the acid alkaline balance diet. The optimal alkaline diet should consist of 80% alkaline foods. You need an alkaline meal plan that will raise your pH level if it is on the lower side. This will mean eating more of the alkaline foods and reducing the acid-forming foods.

We can group the foods as follows:

Highest acidic foods

Chocolate, cheese, homogenized milk, wheat, wheat products, peanuts, walnuts, pasta, pastries, beef, pork, blackberries, cranberries, ice-cream, soft drinks and beer among others.

Lower acidic foods

Coffee, corn, white rice, white and brown sugar, cashews, lima beans, navy beans and pinto beans, oats, lamb, chicken, turkey, potatoes and rhubarb among others.

Least acidic foods

Corn oil, kidney beans and string beans, plums, processed honey, eggs, yoghurt, butter and tea.

Highest alkaline foods

These are lemon, lime, papaya, mango, watermelon, grapefruit, onion, raw spinach, asparagus, broccoli, garlic, herbal teas and olive oil among others.

Lower alkaline foods

Apples, almonds, pears, melon, blueberries, okra, green tea, grapes, kiwis, flaxseed oil, zucchini, beet, celery, green beans, squash, lettuce, sweet potato, dates, figs and maple syrup among others.

Least alkaline foods

These are avocados, oranges, raw honey, bananas, peaches, carrot, cabbage, peas, tofu, amaranth millet, chestnuts, pineapple, quinoa and ginger tea among others.

The following is sample Alkaline meal plan that you can follow to ensure that your body remains healthy!

Keep in mind that you may mix and match the plan as required.

Most new comers tend to follow the 80/20 plan where an individual is required to make a diet that is comprised of 80% alkaline foods and 20% acidic foods.

So the choice lies completely on you!

Day 1

Breakfast: Pumpkin Soup + Zesty Lemon Detox Tea (see recipe at the end of this section)

- Pumpkin, coconut milk, allspice, cinnamon, fresh ginger, sweet potato

Snack Almond Milk

Lunch: Cauliflower Rice with Peas

- Cauliflower, cold-pressed olive oil, oregano, basil, parsley, green peas, salt and pepper

Dinner: Raw Pad Thai

- See recipe at the end of this section

Day 2

Breakfast: Spinach Frittata + Zesty Lemon Detox Tea

- See recipe at the end of the section

Snack: Vegetable and Green Smoothie

- Kale, green apple, tomato, spinach, almond milk, ginger

Lunch: Zucchini Spaghetti with Wild Garlic Pesto

- See recipe at the end of this section

Dinner: Tuna Steaks with Green Salad

- Wild fresh tuna, salt, pepper, lemon, cold pressed olive oil, kale arugula, red onion

Day 3

Breakfast: Mexican Scrambled Eggs + Zesty Lemon Detox Tea

- Eggs, bell peppers, fresh salsa, onion, avocado oil

Snack: Kale Chips

- Kale, cold pressed olive oil, salt, pepper

Lunch: Cauliflower Rice with Peas

- Cauliflower, cold-pressed olive oil, oregano, basil, parsley, green peas, salt and pepper

Dinner: Leek and Sweet Potato Soup

- Leeks, garlic, onion, cold pressed olive oil, coconut milk, Italian seasoning, sweet potato, cinnamon

Day 4

Breakfast: Broccoli Soup + Zesty Lemon Detox Tea

- Avocado oil, broccoli, coconut milk, garlic, onion, sweet potato, broccoli, celery seeds, salt and pepper

Snack: Fresh Tomato Salsa with Alkaline Corn Chips

Lunch: Chickpea Salad

- Chickpeas, roasted red peppers, red onion, cucumber, cold pressed olive oil, Italian seasoning, salt, pepper

Dinner: Gazpacho

- See recipe at the end of this section

Day 5

Breakfast: Mexican Scrambled Eggs + Zesty Lemon Detox Tea

- Eggs, bell peppers, fresh salsa, onion, avocado oil

Snack: Kale Chips

- Kale, cold pressed olive oil, salt, pepper

Lunch: Zucchini Spaghetti with Wild Garlic Pesto

- Zucchini, avocado oil, avocado, garlic pesto (see recipe at the end of this section)

Dinner: Leek and Sweet Potato Soup

- Leeks, garlic, onion, cold pressed olive oil, coconut milk, Italian seasoning, sweet potato, cinnamon

Day 6

Breakfast: Pumpkin Soup + Zesty Lemon Detox Tea

- Pumpkin, coconut milk, allspice, cinnamon, fresh ginger, sweet potato

Snack: Almond Milk

Lunch: Cauliflower Rice with Peas

- Cauliflower, cold-pressed olive oil, oregano, basil, parsley, green peas, salt and pepper

Dinner: Raw Pad Thai

- See recipe after meal plan section

Day 7

Breakfast: Spinach Frittata + Zesty Lemon Detox Tea

- See recipe at the end of this section

Snack: Vegetable Green Smoothie

- Kale, green apple, tomato, spinach, almond milk, ginger

Lunch: Gazpacho

- See recipe after meal plan section

Dinner: Salmon Steak With Kale salad—Lemon juice and sea salt and black pepper

- Salmon, dill, lemon, kale, cucumber, red wine vinaigrette, red onion, roasted red pepper

Day 8

Breakfast: Non-Dairy Coconut Yogurt Apple Parfait

- Coconut yogurt, red apples, cinnamon, oats

Lunch: Avocado Wrap

- Grilled asparagus, whole wheat wrap, avocado, roasted red peppers, balsamic vinegar

Dinner: Broccoli Soup

- Avocado oil, broccoli, coconut milk, garlic, onion, sweet potato, broccoli, celery seeds, salt and pepper

Day 9

Breakfast: Berry Almond Butter Smoothie

- Almond milk, almond butter, blueberries, blackberries

Lunch: Kale and Cucumber Kimchi

- ½ c. prepared kimchi, salt pepper, cucumber, sesame oil

Dinner: Whole Grain Pasta with Kale Pesto

- Use whole grain pasta, see below pesto recipe and substitute kale for ½ of the basil

Day 10

Breakfast: Oats with Apple and Almond Butter

- Rolled oats, granny smith apple, almond butter

Lunch: Balsamic Tuna Salad with Cherry Tomatoes

- Cherry tomatoes, balsamic vinegar, canned tuna, garlic, spinach, kale, salt, pepper.

Dinner: Warm Avocado and Quinoa Salad

- Kale, avocado oil, garbanzo beans, lemon, ginger, garlic, fresh avocado

Day 11

Breakfast: Berry Almond Butter Smoothie

- Almond milk, almond butter, blueberries, blackberries

Lunch: Kale and Cucumber Kimchi

- ½ c. prepared kimchi, salt pepper, cucumber, sesame oil

Dinner: Pasta with Kale Pesto

- Use whole grain pasta, see below pesto recipe and substitute kale for ½ of the basil

Day 12

Breakfast: Non-Dairy Apple Parfait

- Coconut yogurt, red apples, sliced, cinnamon, oats

Lunch: Savory Avocado Wrap

- Grilled asparagus, whole wheat wrap, avocado, roasted red peppers, balsamic vinegar

Dinner: Thai Coconut Broccoli Soup

- Avocado oil, broccoli, coconut milk, garlic, onion, sweet potato, broccoli, celery seeds, salt and pepper

Day 13

Breakfast: Oats with Apple and Almond Butter

- Rolled oats, granny smith apple, almond butter

Lunch: Balsamic Tuna Salad with Cherry Tomatoes

- Cherry tomatoes, balsamic vinegar, canned tuna, garlic, spinach, kale, salt, pepper.

Dinner: Warm Avocado and Quinoa Salad with lemon and ginger

- Kale, avocado oil, garbanzo beans, lemon, ginger, garlic, fresh avocado

Day 14

Breakfast: Berry Almond Butter Smoothie

- Almond milk, almond butter, blueberries, blackberries

Lunch: Kale and Cucumber Kimchi

- ½ c. prepared kimchi, salt pepper, cucumber, sesame oil

Dinner: Pasta with Kale Pesto

- Use whole grain pasta, see below pesto recipe and substitute kale for ½ of the basil

Some specialists recommend that beginners should start the diet with two alkaline meals (breakfast and lunch) and a late dinner. This meal plan involves three 3 alkaline meals a day – breakfast, lunch, and dinner. Some of the recipes may contain processed ingredients, dairy, etc. As I mentioned in the previous chapter, the Alkaline Diet is about balance. There is nothing wrong with consuming a few acidic ingredients every now and then. Some days will be repeated in order for the diet process to be as economic and convenient for you as possible

Sample Recipes for Meal Plan:

The meals listed in the meal plan are just ideas to give you an idea of how you should be eating when eating alkaline. To find specific recipes, there are many alkaline communities, Facebook groups, blogs and websites that offer many free recipes. I've included some sample recipes from the meal plan below to give you an idea.

Turmeric Ginger Lemon Detox Tea

- 2 ½ cups of filtered water
- 1 inch of fresh organic turmeric
- 1 inch of fresh organic ginger root
- pinch of black pepper
- 1 lemon slice (do not boil, add to tea before serving)

Wild Garlic Pesto

- 3 cups chopped fresh basil
- 1 cup chopped spinach
- 1 cup extra virgin olive oil
- 1/2 cup pine nuts
- 2/3 cup grated Parmesan cheese
- 4 tablespoons minced garlic

Raw Pad Thai

- 2 zucchinis, julienne or spiraled
- 2 carrots
- 1 head red cabbage, thinly sliced

- 1 red bell pepper, thinly sliced
- 1/2 cup bean sprouts
- 3/4 cup raw almond butter
- 2 oranges, juiced
- 2 tablespoons raw honey
- 1 tablespoon minced fresh ginger
- 1 tablespoon raw soy sauce
- 1 clove garlic, minced
- 1/4 teaspoon cayenne pepper

Gazpacho

- 2 cups tomatoes, chopped
- 1 small cucumber
- 1 red pepper
- 1 onion
- 2 cloves of garlic
- 1 small chili
- 1 quart of water (preferably alkaline water)
- 4 tbsp. cold-pressed olive oil
- Juice of one fresh lemon
- 1 dash of cayenne pepper
- Sea salt to taste

Spinach Frittata:

- 1 tablespoon avocado oil
- 1 onion
- 4 cups spinach
- 2 cloves garlic, minced
- 8 eggs, (cage free)
- 1/2 teaspoon smoked paprika
- Salt and pepper

Shopping Lists

The alkaline diet is almost completely vegetarian, and even almost vegan because Dairy products are drastically reduced in this diet. This diet also excludes wheat products, which makes is ideal for individuals who live a gluten- free lifestyle and want to cut back on starches. Including the restriction of wheat, the alkaline diet also limits most other major triggers for allergies: milk, walnuts, fish, eggs, peanuts, etc. The alkaline diet focuses on planning your meals to be mostly made up of vegetables and fruits; and while this may sound like an easy change of pace, the transition of altering your normal diet can prove to be significantly challenging. As you begin your transformation to alkaline, refer to the following crucial tips to help make this lifestyle shift easier.

Buy Organic When Possible

Whenever you have the opportunity, you should try to buy organic alkaline foods. While it may seem like a silly and unnecessary splurge, experts have expressed that when eating an alkaline diet, the type of soil your produce was grown in does affect the alkalization of the food. Studies have shown that the type of soil plants grow in can greatly influence their mineral and vitamin content; meaning that not all alkaline food products are equal.

Knowing the Alkalinity of Soil

While the type of soil your produce is grown in is important when purchasing groceries, the acidity of various soils is not common knowledge. The ideal pH level for soil in regards to the number of essential nutrients in the produce is between 6 and 7. Acidic soils that have a pH of lower than six have reduced magnesium and calcium, while soil with a pH higher than 7 may have chemically insufficient manganese, zinc, iron, and copper.

Drink Alkaline Water

You don't have to just rely on alkaline foods to help your body reduce acidity; there is alkaline water and even pH drops available to help increase your intake. Alkaline water contains a pH of 9 to 11. While distilled water is still fine to drink, using a reverse osmosis filter can cause it to become slightly acidic. If you cannot find bottle alkaline water, you can always add pH drops, lemon, lime, or baking soda to purified bottled water to increase alkalinity.

Complete Alkaline Diet Grocery List

You already know that an alkaline diet restricts your intake of sugar and processed foods; so, what can you eat? To help make your transition into the alkaline lifestyle that much easier, here is a complete list of the top alkaline foods that you can eat while on the diet:

<u>Fresh Fruits and Vegetables</u>
Alfalfa
Alfalfa sprouts
Artichokes
Asparagus (green tips)
Avocado
Bamboo shoots
Banana
Beans
Beets
Bell Peppers
Broccoli
White Cabbage
Carrots
Cauliflower
Celery
Chard
Chayote
Chicory
Chives
Collard Greens
Cucumbers
Dandelions
Dills
Endives
Garlic Greens
Ginger
Grapefruit
Horseradish
Kale
Leek
Lemon
Lime
Lettuce
Black Olives
Onion
Parsley
Parsnips
Peas
Pumpkin
Radish

Raspberry
Spinach
Sprouts (all)
Summer squash
Swiss chard
Tomatoes
Turnips
Watermelon
Wheat Grass
Zucchini

<u>Legumes</u>
Lentils
Lima Beans
White Beans

<u>Beverages</u>
Water
Coconut Water

<u>Fats/ Oils</u>
Flaxseed Oil
Olive Oil
Sesame Oil

<u>Dairy Products</u>
Goats Milk
Goats Cheese

<u>Bread/ Grains</u>
Sprouted Bread
Spelt Bread
Quinoa
Spelt Pasta

<u>Nuts and Seeds</u>
Almonds
Cumin Seeds
Pumpkin Seeds
Fennel Seeds
Flaxseed

Chai Seeds
Sesame Seeds

Vegetable Oil
Canola oil
Sunflower Oil
Corn oil

Foods to Avoid on an Alkaline Diet

Meat/Poultry/Sea food
Veal
Lamb
Beef
Chicken
Duck
Fish
Oysters
Turkey
Crab
Lobster
Goose
Pork
Clams

Condiments
Jams and Jellies
Vinegar
Ketchup
Mustard
Mayonnaise

Breads/Flours
Cereals
Corn
Cornstarch
Pasta
Rye Bread
Rye Flour
White Bread
Whole Grain Bread

Fats/ Oils
Margarine
Butter

Dairy Products
Milk
Butter
Cheese
Eggs

Beverages
Liquor
Soft Drinks
Wine
Black Tea
Beer
Coffee
Processed Juices
Sport drinks

Fruits/Vegetables
Preserved Fruits
Preserved Vegetables
Canned Fruits
Glazed Fruits
Processed Veggies
Canned Olives
Pickled Vegetables

Nuts/Seeds
Cashews
Peanuts
Roasted Nuts
Salted Nuts
Walnuts

Grains/Legumes
Brown rice
White rice

Sweets/ Desserts
Artificial sweeteners
Malt Sugar
All dessert products
Molasses
Sugar—
Refined

Cane   Brown Sugar
Beet Sugar

Additional Habits that Cause Acidity in the Body

- Alcohol and Drug Use
- Frequent Caffeine Consumption
- Overuse of Antibiotics
- Chronic Stress and Worry
- Lack of Exercise
- Over Exercising
- Lack of Dietary Fiber
- Excess Meat Consumption
- Pesticides and Herbicides
- Shallow Breathing
- Food Colorings and Preservatives
- Excess Hormones in Foods, Beauty and Bath Products, and Plastics
- Over- Exposure to Chemicals and Radiation

Conclusion

I thank you for purchasing this book and we hope this marks the start of a breakthrough in your wellness journey. Embarking on your Alkaline Adventure can be scary and overwhelming at first. I hope I've been able to help provide you with practical steps and tips for making this transition easier.

As I've expressed in the book, it's better to start little by little. Take baby steps instead of trying to launch full-force into this diet. Since this diet is meant to be more of a long-term lifestyle change, the last thing you want to do is burn yourself out too soon. It may be as simple as trying to start by eliminating excess sugar from your diet, and introduce more vegetables. From there, you can continue to eliminate problem acid foods and continue augmenting with vegetables and alkaline substitutes.

As you progress, you'll see very real results in your well-being and the way you feel, and it will be just the motivation you need to forge ahead. The most important thing you can do at that point is to make it your own. Many people make the mistake of trying to follow diet books and guides to a T. The problem with this approach is that everyone's body is different and everyone's eating habits, motivations, and patterns are slightly unique. If you can make the alkaline diet your own, and approach it with your own unique style, you'll find it much easier to stay committed.

I want to leave you with one thought: eating well is about being kind to ourselves. We are being gentle with our bodies, treating our bodies with the respect and gravity they deserve. After all, we only get one body, and it is our vehicle that will carry us down all the roads of life to our final destination. Anyone who has actually taken the trouble to read this book already understands this to some degree. You care about your health and your body and that's why you want to preserve it, and treat it with kindness. I applaud you for taking the necessary steps to get to this point. You are already miles ahead of most other people. One step at a time we will help each other forge ahead on our wellness journey.

One step at a time, we will overcome obstacle after obstacle until wellness is in our grasp.

Best wishes to you and thank you for taking the first step!

--Felicia